Enrolled Nurse
CONVERSION PROGRAMME 1

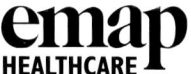

First edition 1993.
Reprinted 1995, 1997.
This revised edition, 1998.
Reprinted 1999, 2000.

Published by
Emap Healthcare
Greater London House
London NW1 7EJ.

Companies and representatives throughout the world

Printed in Great Britain by
Drogher Press
Christchurch, Dorset

ISBN 1–902499–05–0

Revision 1998

Editorial Team

Andrea Cassidy, writer; lecturer, School of Health Studies, University of Bradford

Patsy Dale, chief sub-editor, Emap Healthcare Open Learning

Joan Henriques, writer; editorial associate, Cambridge Training and Development Ltd

Cathy Hull, editor, Emap Healthcare Open Learning

Antonia Tully, writer; editor, Cambridge Training and Development Ltd

Ann Winter, writer; tutor, School of Health Studies, University of Bradford

Critical Readers

Jane Darke, healthcare consultant

Liz Jacques, open learning programme leader, Department of Health Studies, University of York

Nancy Jane Lee, tutor, Department of Nursing, University of Salford

Edel Mullen, course director, open learning, School of Nursing and Midwifery, Queens University, Belfast

Hema Mungar, programme director, School of Midwifery and Health Visiting, University of Manchester

Annie Persaud, health lecturer, Division of Health Studies, University of Bradford

Neil Snee, director of nursing and quality, Medway NHS Trust

Karen Staniland, open learning conversion programme leader, Department of Nursing, University of Salford

Student Testers

Janet Hutchinson, sister, Cottingley Hall Nursing Home, Bingley; community nurse, Bradford District

Lis Krzykawski, staff nurse, Bradford Royal Infirmary

Julia Layzell, junior sister, Horsham Hospital

Andrea Migasiuk, enrilled nurse, intensive care department, Princess Elizabeth Hospital, Guernsey

Design and Production

Claire Conway, senior designer, Emap Healthcare

Yvonne Dunne, layout artist

Julie Edwards, projects production controller, Emap Healthcare

Graham Ogilvie, head of creative services, Emap Healthcare

Destine Simon, projects manager, Emap Healthcare Open Learning

Andrew Sumner, production manager, Emap Healthcare

Photographs

Laurence Bulaitis, photographer

Sue Lloyd, picture researcher, *Nursing Times*

Louise Thomas, picture researcher, *Health Service Journal*

Special thanks to Medway NHS Trust for the use of their hospital as a photographic resource.

Reading List

Moya Davis, open and distance learning consultant and author

PREVIOUS CREDITS

The Authors

John Adams, nurse teacher, Sir Gordon Roberts College of Nursing and Midwifery, Kettering General Hospital: P2.

Brian Booth, assistant clinical editor, *Nursing Times*: P5

Philip Burnard, director of postgraduate nursing studies, University of Wales College of Medicine, Cardiff: P6

Moya Davis, distance learning consultant: P1, P3, P4

John Hiley, head of business development, University of Central Lancashire: M1

Sandra Lask, part-time lecturer in psychology: P7

Derek Ormerod, partner at Systech Training Systems Development, Preston: Foundation

Kate Robinson, dean of the Faculty of Health Care and Social Studies, Luton College of Higher Education; formerly chair of nursing development and lecturer in health and social studies, Open university: R1, R2, R3

Barbara Scammell, training consultant: Foundation

Editors

Lynn Earnshaw, educational design consultant

Pamela Shakespeare, lecturer in health and social welfare, Open University

Members of the Steering Committee

Pat Darcy, formerly director of nurse education, Western Area College of Nursing, Londonderry, Northern Ireland

Moya Davis, distance learning consultant and author

Lynn Earnshaw, educational design consultant

Jill Fardell, formerly open learning editor, *Nursing Times* Open Learning Programme

Sue Frost, formerly head of school, School of Health Studies, University of Portsmouth

Margaret Johnson, tutor, clinical education and practice, John Radcliffe Infirmary, Oxford

Jean Lowe, formerly English National Board; education officer to the programme

Anne Palmer, formerly principal lecturer, South Bank University, London

Marianne Phillips, formerly programme co-ordinator, *Nursing Times* Open Learning Programme

Bob Price, formerly vice-principal/lecturer in cancer nursing, Royal Marsden Hospital, London

Kate Robinson, dean, Faculty of Health Care and Social Studies, Luton College of Higher Education; formerly chair of nursing development and lecturer in health and social studies, Open University

Ann Ryall-Davies, formerly director of professional services, Welsh National Board

Chris Wakeling, formerly director of nurse education, Highland College of Nursing and Midwifery, Inverness

Mary Waltham, formerly editorial director, Macmillan Magazines Limited

Contents

INTRODUCTION

Term 1

Foundation: Responding to Change

R1   Nursing: A Research-based Profession
   (i)   Research and the cycle of learning and practice

P1   Health and Illness
   (i)   A personal view of health and illness
   (ii)   Health and power
   (iii)   Professionals and consumers

P2   Human Biography
   (i)   A personal approach
   (ii)   Different lives, different perspectives

Term 2

P3   Human Environment
   (i)   Public health and personal health
   (ii)   Organising the nation's health

R2   Focusing on Research Knowledge
   (i)   Sources of knowledge
   (ii)   Rubbing shoulders with research
   (iii)   Reading research reports

P4   Nursing Competency
   (i)   What is a registered nurse?
   (ii)   The competences in context
   (iii)   Acquiring level-1 competences

M1   Principles of Management
   (i)   Are you a manager?
   (ii)   How do you manage?

Term 3

P5   Client Assessment

    (i)   Assessment in context

    (ii) Client assessment in practice

P6   Facilitating Learning

    (i)   Learning and communication

    (ii) The process of facilitation

P7   Health Promotion

    (i)   Health promotion: a question of choice?

    (ii) Issues and dilemmas

    (iii) Planning a health promotion programme

R3   Research Approaches

    (i)   Ways of seeing

    (ii) The view from above: experiments and surveys

    (iii) The view from within: ethnography and phenomenology

Introduction

These materials will support your learning on the Emap Healthcare Open Learning enrolled nurse conversion programme. They include:

- **The Profile Pack**
- *A Student's Guide To Open Learning,* **by Moya Davis**
- **Student Notes**
- **Learning Materials: 1 (This book)**
- **Learning Materials: 2**
- **Three specialist modules:**   *Community Health Care*

    Care of the Mother and Newborn

    Mental Health and Learning Disabilities

The materials are only part of the support you are given. You will also have access to a tutor/counsellor and a practice supervisor, who should stay with you, and support you throughout your studies.

Most students find that open learning is a new experience, and they want to get a feel for what it means from the start. You might find it useful, therefore, to begin by reading The Profile Pack and *A Student's Guide to Open Learning,* and to start developing your own profile. It is also a good idea to make contact with your tutor and to find out about the systems and resources which have been established to support your study.

Once you have done this, you can begin to plan your work. Remember: you can take as much or as little time to complete the Activities as you feel you need. They are designed to help you work at a pace and a time to suit your own needs.

The programme materials are regularly updated and you will find them relevant to your current practice. As part of the revision process many past students have suggested improvements, based on their experience of completing the programme. Our tutors, too, have offered advice. Each time we revise, therefore, the materials become richer and enhanced in some way.

A note about reflection

Many of the Activities throughout the book encourage you to keep a diary. You will find more guidance on using a professional diary in The Profile Pack. It is important that part of your diary is kept private — for your eyes only — so that you can be completely honest about what you think. Remember, though, that if you are writing about clients or other colleagues, the diary is confidential, and you do not need to show it to anyone else.

Some Activities ask you to pause for a moment and think about certain questions. Again, these will be your private thoughts, and you may wish to jot them down in your diary as well. These are important Activities as they will help you work out your own views — so try not to skip them.

ACTIVITY 1
diary
Write a definition of good health that could be applied to anyone in the world.

1

WORK PLANNER

At the beginning of each Section there is a Work Planner which will give you a brief outline of what is included, and help you to organise your work. Some Activities ask you to do practical things, which you may not be able to complete at the time you are working through that particular Section. Spend a few minutes at the beginning of your work on each Section checking the Work Planner and planning how you are going to make any necessary arrangements for practical work.

Essential reading

Some Activities ask you to refer to other literature. This essential reading is part of the learning programme, and you should make every effort to find the material required.

FOCUS

At the end of each piece of work there is a FOCUS Activity, which helps you to draw together the ideas and situations you have been exploring, and to relate them to your own experience. This will almost certainly involve some written work. It is a good idea to keep your written work in a folder so that you can refer back to it as your work progresses.

Notes

Keeping notes and jotting down your ideas is an important part of the learning process. You can do this by writing formal notes as you read new literature or discuss ideas with your tutor. Your profile should also provide you with space to tease out new ideas, and to work through your own thoughts and feelings. You will also find space on the pages of these materials for you to respond to what has been written, or to brainstorm some ideas. Remember: don't feel apprehensive about writing on the materials — they have been designed with this in mind.

Choosing which Section to study

The materials are divided into six terms. Between four and five new topics are introduced each term, each of which will introduce you to research, management and professional development issues. They can, however, be adapted to suit your own learning needs. You might, for instance, use topics from across Sections of the whole programme to complete an essay or research. Remember: the material is there to support you, and it is up to you to use it to your best advantage.

Keeping in touch

We hope you enjoy working through these materials. If you would like to tell us about your experience of the programme — good or bad — we would like to hear from you. Our address is: Emap Healthcare Open Learning, Emap Healthcare, Greater London House, Hampstead Road, London NW1 7EJ.

Other Emap Healthcare Open Learning materials

Throughout this book we refer to other Emap Healthcare Open Learning (formerly Macmillan Open Learning) materials you might find useful. Here is a list of specific titles available for you to sample at a specially reduced price:

- The Ethics, Practice and Safety of Complementary Therapies
- Groups and Group Processes in Professional Relationships
- Planning and Carrying out an Enquiry
- Health Care and Information
- Why Evaluate Health Care?
- Caring and Health
- Health Promotion Strategies
- Getting Across the Message About Health Care

Each of these units has been taken from one of eight modules from our BSc (Hons) Professional Practice in Health Care and is also available for purchase. The titles are as follows:

- Enquiring Into Healthcare Practice
- Complementary Therapies and Healthcare Practice
- Professional Relationships: Influences on health care
- Health Care and the Information Age
- Healthcare Evaluation
- Values and the Person: Ideas that influence health care
- Health Promotion in Professional Practice
- Influences in Health Care: Media perspectives

For more information about all Emap Healthcare Open Learning materials contact:

Emap Healthcare Open Learning
Emap Healthcare
Greater London House
Hampstead Road
London
NW1 7EJ
Telephone: 020 7874 0600
Fax: 020 7874 0601
E-mail: open.learning@healthcare.emap.co.uk

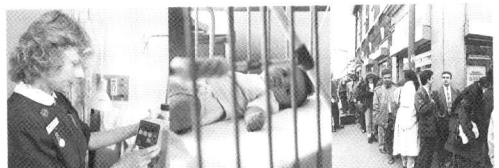

Term 1

The Sections which make up the first term's work focus on individuals' beliefs and attitudes about healthcare and nursing. In the Foundation Section we ask you to explore your own thoughts about the two central themes of this programme: change in the nursing profession, and your role in it.

In Section R1 we look at some of the myths surrounding research. It will help you to understand the nature of research-based knowledge and its implications for your practice. We also introduce you to evidence-based practice.

The next two Sections, (P1 and P2), explore individual ideas about health and illness, and ask you to consider how your own views may differ from those of other groups in society, and the impact these differences may have on the relationship between healthcare organisations, nurses and clients.

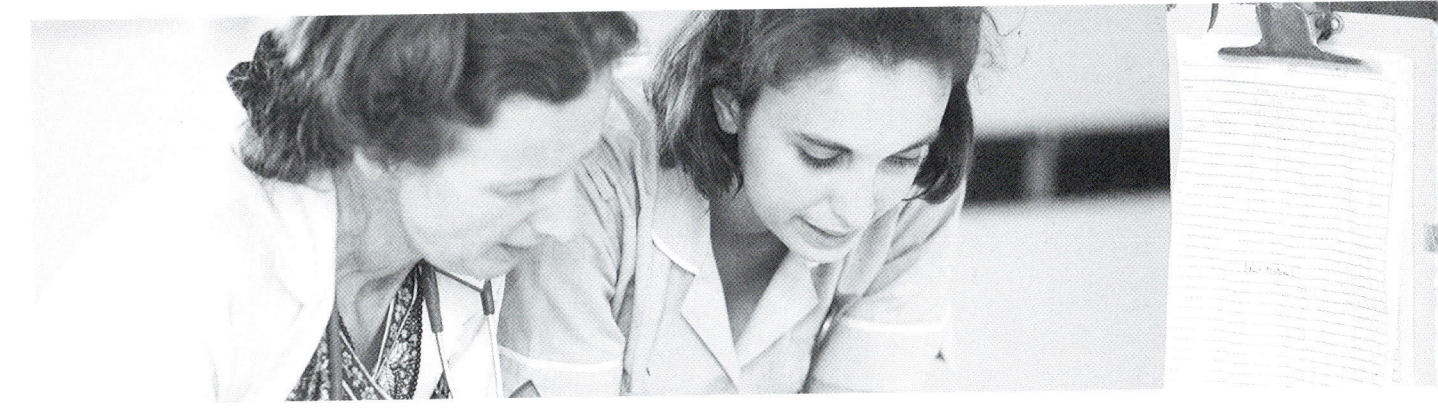

Responding to change

Nursing is used to coping with change, but in recent years managing change has become part of everyday life. This first Section includes some of the factors responsible for the current climate of change:

- The Government White Papers
- Project 2000.

You are asked in this Part to explore your feelings about the nursing profession and about yourself as a nurse. In looking at some of the pressures for change, you may clarify your thoughts about how some of the changes will affect you now and in the future.

You will also look at your new role in becoming a student again and consider:

- The other people in your life and how this will affect them
- Practical steps to make time in your week for this study.

GETTING STARTED ON THIS PROGRAMME

Welcome to the EMAP Healthcare Open Learning enrolled nurse conversion programme. We hope you will find the work challenging, stimulating and, above all, enjoyable.

The focus of your work on this programme will be you, both as an individual and as a member of the nursing profession. Using the Profile Pack which accompanies these materials, you have begun a process of change and self-development which will continue throughout your nursing career.

Remember that before you start work on this programme, you should have read through all the support materials in your student pack. You should also make sure you have read *A Student's Guide to Open Learning* (see the Introductionto this book, page 3).

The programme is designed on the assumption that you can do it with the support of a trained tutor/counsellor, a supervisor from your own workplace and a programme co-ordinator at EMAP Healthcare Open Learning.

Do not forget, though, that you are the most important learning resource on the programme. Your life and work experience, and the sense you have made of them, are unique, and the work you do on this programme will build and develop on this in a way that is unique to you.

WORK PLANNER

For this Section you need to be familiar with the basics of:

1. GOVERNMENT WHITE PAPERS

    (i)   *Caring for People*, Command Paper 849, 1989[†]

    (ii) *Working for Patients*, Command Paper 555, 1989[†]

    (iii) *The New NHS: Modern, Dependable*, Command Paper 3807, 1997[†]

2. PROJECT 2000

    (i)   *Counting the Cost*, Project paper 8, February 1987[*]

    (ii) *The Final Proposals*, Project paper 9, February 1987[*]

    (iii) *The Facts About Project 2000*, press release, May 21, 1988 (the government's response to the proposals)[*]

[†] Available from The Stationery Office, PO Box 276, London SW8 5DT; tel: 0171 873 0011. (Telephone first for price.)
[*] Available from the UKCC, 23 Portland Place, London W1N 3AF; tel. 0171 637 7181

ACTIVITY 1
diary
For your first Activity, we would like you to ask yourself two questions: 'Why did I become a nurse?' and 'Why did I choose to train as an EN?' Jot down your answers in your diary — you can be as honest and as open as you want, because no one is going to see your answers except you.

FEEDBACK

Among your reasons for becoming a nurse, we guess that almost all of you would have put something about caring for others, maybe people with special needs, but did you give any other, perhaps more private, reasons as well? Did you want a career in which you knew that people would depend on you? Did you have ambitions to be a doctor but failed to get the necessary academic qualifications? Did you just want to get away and do something interesting?

Whatever else you wrote down, you might have included a statement about the status of nursing in society which attracted you. We'll come back to this idea in a minute.

Now the second part of Activity 1. If you are an EN, why did you choose the shorter training period? Was it because the academic entry requirements were lower, with the emphasis on practical nursing skills? Whatever your reasons, your qualifications have served you and the health service well in the years since you qualified, and many aspects of your work will have been both rewarding and worthwhile.

SO WHY THE NEED FOR CHANGE?

The government's changes have enormous implications for the way in which nursing care is provided, demanding greater flexibility and broader skills from all nurses. But these are not new ideas. The nursing profession recognised as far back as the early 1970s that nurses would be meeting new challenges from the 1990s onwards, challenges brought about by social and political changes. Some of these challenges have been precipitated by *demographic* changes (changes in the way society is structured), including:

*   Fewer school leavers to meet recruitment needs

*   People living longer, but not necessarily in better health

*   More working women.

Political changes, such as Britain's involvement in the European Union (EU), have also created pressure for change. Free movement between member countries of the EU means that regulations for education of healthcare professionals have had to be more standardised than they were in the past.

The Government White Papers

ACTIVITY 2
diary
Now think about the current state of healthcare and the nursing profession. Write down some of the changes in the years since you qualified. How have these changes affected you and the way you feel about nursing?

Change in the National Health Service has become a major political issue. In January 1989, the government issued the White Paper *Working for Patients*[1], which proposed major changes in the way the health service was managed. The emphasis was on providing a more cost-effective service and giving the consumer greater choice in who provides care and where it is provided.

The White Paper also proposed that those hospitals which were being managed efficiently should become self-governing. Those that did so were able to set their own pay levels and conditions of service for their staff.

There was considerable opposition to the White Paper from the healthcare professions. The Royal College of Nursing and the British Medical Association, in particular, mounted major campaigns against the proposals. Their members believed that the proposals paved the way to privatising the health service, a move which would lead to a two-tier health system which would further disadvantage the most vulnerable in society[2].

A second White Paper, *Caring for People*[3], also published in 1989, set out the government's proposals for community care. When the recommendations of this paper were implemented, more care was provided within the community, and responsibility for much of this care shifted from the health service to the social services. Community nursing was seen as central to these proposals, but the shift in emphasis from health care to social care suggested that this, too, was to undergo some major changes.

In December 1997 the Labour government published *The New NHS: Modern, Dependable*[4]. This White Paper aims to end the internal market and to reverse the 'command and control' policies of the 1970s. Its goal is to encourage local responsibility, and partnership is seen as the key to achieving this — co-operation will replace competition. There will be an end to two-tier GP fundholding, giving all GPs the same amount of influence.

NHS trusts will now be properly accountable and it will be the responsibility of every trust board to promote clinical excellence and quality. The Commission for Health Improvement will ensure that health issues are tackled at a local level and shortcomings addressed. The emphasis in this White Paper is on performance management going beyond costs and volume to patients, including outcome, health gain and patient experience.

ACTIVITY 3
knowledge base
Look through, or ask your tutor or mentor about, whichever of the White Papers — *Working for Patients, Caring for People* or *The New NHS: Modern, Dependable* — is most relevant to your own area of work. Aim to get a general idea of the contents, rather than to absorb every word. Summarise the key points of the White Paper you selected.

FEEDBACK

The first two White Papers related to healthcare professions in general, but had particular significance for nurses in two important respects:

- The emphasis on cost-effectiveness in the health service (presented in *Working for Patients*)

- The move towards providing more care in the community, with shorter hospital stays and the prevention of ill health (outlined in *Caring for People*).

The New NHS: Modern, Dependable emphasises the move towards provider performance management and local accountability.

Project 2000

The United Kingdom Central Council (UKCC), formed in 1983, had to take account of European directives when formulating its rules for the education and training of nurses. In 1986, the UKCC's proposals for the preparation of nurses were announced —proposals which came to be known as Project 2000. Project 2000 was about determining what was needed to make nurses more suitably qualified to do their job in the future.

A number of reports on the education needs of nurses were commissioned and studied by the profession before the UKCC proposals were finally accepted.

As far back as 1970, a committee, under the chairmanship of Professor Asa Briggs, was set up to 'review the role of the nurse and the midwife in the hospital and the community and the education required for that role, so that the best use is made of available manpower to meet present needs and the needs of an integrated health service'[5]. The recommendations of this committee (The Briggs Report) were not implemented.

In 1985, the Judge Report, following the investigations of another committee commissioned by the Royal College of Nursing, recommended that nurses had the 'right to an education which will equip them to question as well as obey, to discover as well as to be taught, to learn from those who have never been nurses as well as those who have been excellent ones'[6].

The registered practitioner as defined by Project 2000 was expected to be more autonomous and adaptable, and able to work in any setting, institution or community.

ACTIVITY 4
discussion
After some careful thought, make some notes about what you think Project 2000 is saying to you. How do you feel about this? How effective is Project 2000 in developing confident, practice-based nurses? Discuss some of your notes with your supervisor, even if you do not want to say exactly how you feel.

FEEDBACK

It is interesting that both the Briggs and Judge reports recognised the difficulties being experienced by enrolled nurses whose career prospects were poor and, according to Judge, 'although ENs were to be trained to assist the first-level nurse in her work, they were in fact used interchangeably ... with obvious risks to the second-level nurse herself'[6].

Many enrolled nurses regard Project 2000 with mixed feelings. They can recognise that the profession is changing, and that they must change with it, but deep down they see the provisions of Project 2000 as a statement about their own value to the future of nursing.

Of course, as we acknowledged earlier, you know that this is not the case. One of the reasons that this programme came into being was to enable you to build on your valuable experience and knowledge and plan a programme of personal and professional development.

We recognise that you are skilled nurses, many of whom have often fulfilled the role of a first-level nurse. During the programme we will be using the techniques of open learning to explore those aspects of your nursing practice which can be changed to make you into a 'knowledgeable practitioner', and to build on your existing skills in three main areas: research, professional development, and management.

Research: This module does not attempt to make you into mini-researchers. It is simply intended to enable you to understand what you know now, and how you know it; and then to decide, from the variety of research-based evidence available, how to select the most appropriate way to underpin your practice or to implement change.

Professional development: As we said earlier, nurses are working in a changing environment. This module focuses on the political and social influences on the environment in which you and your clients live and work and, in particular, the way in which these influence the way client care is and could be provided.

Management: Everyone, whether actively involved in management or not, possesses management skills which they use in their everyday life and work. Some people's management skills are better developed than others, depending on their life experience. This module will enable you to acknowledge your personal and time management styles and skills; to explore how you apply these in your personal and professional roles — and how to improve them to manage your work, and the resources available for client care, more effectively.

Throughout the programme, we will be asking you to reflect on your existing practice, and to develop your awareness of yourself as a nurse, and as a member of the group — the team of healthcare professionals with whom you work.

THE PROFESSION IS CHANGING – DO YOU WANT TO CHANGE?

ACTIVITY 5
diary
Why did you decide to enrol as a student nurse on the EMAP Healthcare Open Learning programme? Jot down your reasons, and then note down how you feel about returning to study — both positive and negative feelings.

FEEDBACK

It is always a good idea to try to identify your *motives* – the reasons you have for feeling and acting the way you do. Understanding what they are and how they affect you can be a great help, first in planning where you go next, and second in controlling any feelings of anxiety you have about your future.

You might have been motivated to become a student by a number of factors :

- Pressure from your work environment ('I have to change or I'll get left behind')

- A need for improved status ('People will think better of me if I do this') or self-esteem ('I'll feel better about myself if ...)

- The need for material improvement ('This change will give me the opportunity to earn more money').

You may also have seen the opportunities for change as a route to personal growth ('I've got to change to become the person I feel I could be').

Acting against this, you might have noted some negative factors such as fear of change — worries about losing a sense of 'belonging' to friends and colleagues, or about the threat that failure might present to your self-esteem. ('Might I fail?' 'What will people think of me if I don't know the answers to their questions?' and so on.)

In answering Activity 5, you may have found that you came up with conflicting motives — perhaps you recognise the benefits of change, but also worry about the uncertainties such change will bring.

At this point we want to say three things:

- Most people feel threatened by change

- The motives people have for wanting or resisting change are often very complicated

- The EMAP Healthcare Open Learning conversion programme takes both of these factors into account — it is designed to build up your self-esteem, not to threaten it; it will build on what you know, not on what you don't know.

The first enrolled nurse students registered with this conversion programme in 1990. Since that time several thousand students have successfully completed their study. Most students say that, initially, they feel daunted at the prospect of studying, and resentful at the changes being imposed upon them. They quickly move on from this position and become enthusiastic about learning new ideas, at the same time recognising — often for the first time — the extent of their current knowledge and skills:

> 'I used to think I was really stupid, and that learning was for clever people. The conversion programme helped me to realise that I know a lot, and am good at my practice. I'm learning new things all the time. It's great. I just don't want to stop now I've started' — an EN student

BECOMING A STUDENT AGAIN

In the next part of this Foundation Section we ask you to take a close look at your life, to identify the significant people, the roles you play and the expectations other people have of you. All these are important because you will have to make changes to your life in order to fit this open learning programme into it, and these changes will affect other people.

Role-playing

Can you remember the first time you wore your nurse's uniform and met your first patients or clients? For most people, the experience of playing their first professional *role* is just like playing a part in a play.

You can probably remember how self-conscious you felt, maybe even wondering if your clients would take you seriously or perhaps 'see right through' you to the real, nervous you underneath.

If you compare yourself then with the professional you are now, you will almost certainly be amazed at the changes. The self-consciousness has gone. You play your nursing role not as an actor, but as 'you'. The role of the nurse has become a very central part of the image you have when you think about yourself.

This process, first of playing roles and then of making them part of ourselves, part of our own self-image, is at the centre of human development. The roles we have affect the way we see and feel about ourselves. They also affect the way we relate to other people. Understanding the importance of roles and self-image is at the heart of the understanding of all human relationships, not just that between nurse and client[7].

ACTIVITY 6
diary
Make a list in your diary of the significant people in your life, for example, your partner, parents, manager.

Your list probably included all those people who have an important influence on the way you live your life.

ACTIVITY 7
diary
How many major roles do you play in your life? Nursing is obviously one of them, but what others are important to you? For many people, roles such as wife or husband, father or mother, daughter or son, representative or member of a sports team will be significant, but the list you write will be unique to you as an individual. Make a list of the significant roles you feel you play in your life.

You may be surprised just how many different roles you play. The complexities of the roles we all have inevitably make for an interesting life, but before looking at the details of this complexity it is worth making the distinction between:

- Those *social* roles we take on more or less voluntarily — parent, secretary to the neighbourhood watch, a nurse

- Those *biological* roles about which we have no choice, such as being a son or a daughter.

Role Expectations

ACTIVITY 8
diary
Look back to the list of roles you made in Activity 7. Which of them did you take on voluntarily, and which of them did you have no choice about?

The fact that we each play so many roles in life, often roles about which we have no choice, can present us with a number of challenges and problems. One of these lies in the fact that for each role we play, other people have *expectations* of what we must do to play the role properly.

The expectations that *significant others* have of us can cause lots of problems. These problems generally fall into two categories:

- Problems caused when your view of your role is different from that of the significant other

- Problems caused when two or more significant others expect you to behave in ways which conflict.

Role tensions such as these can exist in both the long term and the short term. For example, if you have children you may find they have certain expectations of you as a parent which you do not share. Issues such as who does the housework and shopping are typical long-term 'problems' in family life.

ACTIVITY 9
diary
Think about your home life. Can you spot any areas where the individuals have expectations of your role which you do not share? Jot down your thoughts, noting whether these are long-term or short-term problems.

You may have come up with several examples in answer to Activity 9. Most people experience role tensions of some sort, and most find ways of accommodating them in everyday life.

Your Role as a Student

Being a student is going to introduce a new set of significant people into your life — your tutor/counsellor, for example. If you have not studied recently, you are going to have to establish new priorities to fit your role as a student into all the other roles you currently play.

The best way to illustrate this is to work out how your existing roles fill a typical week.

ACTIVITY 10
action
Look back at the notes you made in Activities 7 and 8. Sketch out a typical working week on a sheet of paper. How much time each day is allocated to each of the roles you listed? You may also want to copy this into your diary, but you will need the sheet for Activity 12.

We estimate that in following the EMAP Healthcare Open Learning conversion programme you will need between six and 12 hours' studying time a week. After looking at your response to Activity 10 you may have decided that something is going to have to move over to make room for your new role.

There is a temptation when faced with a task such as this to try to find all the time needed for study by scrapping some 'voluntary' roles in order to continue to play the other roles without change — and without confronting the expectations other people have about them.

For example, you might find it easier to give up leisure activities than to delegate some responsibilities to others.

To take this line is probably a mistake for most people. Keeping a balance between work, study and recreation is good for you, and if you are happy it will be good for all the people with whom you interact.

Sharing the Decisions

By now, you can see that becoming a student inevitably affects other people in your life.

ACTIVITY 11
diary
Suppose you have decided that some of the study time required for the EMAP Healthcare Open Learning conversion programme must come from time taken by the key roles you currently play. Who is going to be affected, and how?

To avoid at least some of the problems this might cause, it is as well to share the decision-making process with the people who will be most affected.

In the next Activity we suggest a way in which you can work with the significant people in your life to reach a decision you are all happy with.

ACTIVITY 12
action
Choose two or three of the people who will be most affected by your becoming a student again. Spend some time with each of them to look again at Activities 9, 10 and 11. Tell them the responses you gave to Activities 9 and 11 and show them the sketch of your work which you did in Activity 10. Ask them if they agree with the responses you have given. Then take some time to talk about your new role as a student and the adjustments that other people will have to make. The aim of this Activity is to help others see for themselves how your becoming a student will affect both you and them.

FEEDBACK

For many people, the process of sharing decision-making with the significant people in their lives will not be a new idea. If you belong to this group you will know the real support that grows out of the sharing process.

If the idea of talking through the pros and cons of a course of action and then reaching a joint decision is a new one to you, don't be put off from trying.

If you feel you need some guidance in this area, ask your tutor/counsellor, who may be able to organise some role-play sessions to give you practice, which will boost your confidence.

Of course it is important for everyone involved to remember that there are many advantages to following the programme; for example, in many situations:

• Friends and colleagues may be stimulated by your new ideas and knowledge

• Children are often excited at having a 'student' parent with whom to share experiences of learning, and partners take pride in your developing skills and self-confidence, particularly if they feel they are actively involved in the process.

ACTIVITY 13
diary
Make your own list of the advantages to you and to the other people in your life of your following this programme.

SELF-CONFIDENCE

Now you have had the chance to work out some of the practical issues of roles and relationships which are involved in the business of returning to study, there is one more important area to think about. How do *you* feel about becoming a student again?

You will have begun to explore these issues in your early work on the Profile Pack.

You are therefore by now beginning to accept that your existing skills and knowledge, gained from experience, whether in or outside the nursing role, are an important resource for learning. Throughout the programme we will constantly ask you to reflect upon your experience, to organise it and share it with others and to build new knowledge and skills on to it.

Last but not least, remember another important group of individuals who will benefit from the work you do on this programme — the patients and clients with whom you work. They stand to benefit not just from the increased skills and knowledge you will bring to your work, but from your increased self-knowledge and self-confidence. Knowing what makes you tick, psychologically speaking, is an enormous advantage when you try to understand other people and their reactions to sickness and health.

FOCUS

In this Section, *Foundation: Responding to change*, you have identified priorities that are going to change as you become a student, and you have discussed the implications of these changes with other people who will be affected by them. Look back to the 'working week' you sketched out in Activity 10 and redraw it, showing your new timetable and the way you will reorganise your roles and responsibilities to fit your study needs. Indicate those roles you have decided to give up, and those where someone else will take over part of the role for you.

Your tutor will be interested to see this timetable, and to discuss any areas of conflict which you feel remain.

REFERENCES

1   Department of Health. *Working for Patients*. London: HMSO, Cmnd 555, 1989.

2   Turner, T. Counter-attack. *Nursing Times* 1989; **85**: 16, 22.

3   Secretaries of State for Health, Social Security, Wales and Scotland. *Caring for People. Community care in the next decade and beyond*. London: HMSO, Cmnd 849, 1989.

4   Department of Health. *The New NHS: Modern, Dependable*. London: The Stationery Office, Cmnd 3807, 1997.

5   Committee on Nursing. *Report of the Committee on Nursing* (Briggs Report). London: HMSO, Cmnd 5115, 1972.

6   Royal College of Nursing, Commission on Nursing Education. *The Education of Nurses. A new Dispensation* (Judge Report). London: Royal College of Nursing, 1985.

7   Argyle, M. *The Psychology of Interpersonal Behaviour*. Harmondsworth: Penguin, 1983; Chapters 8 and 9.

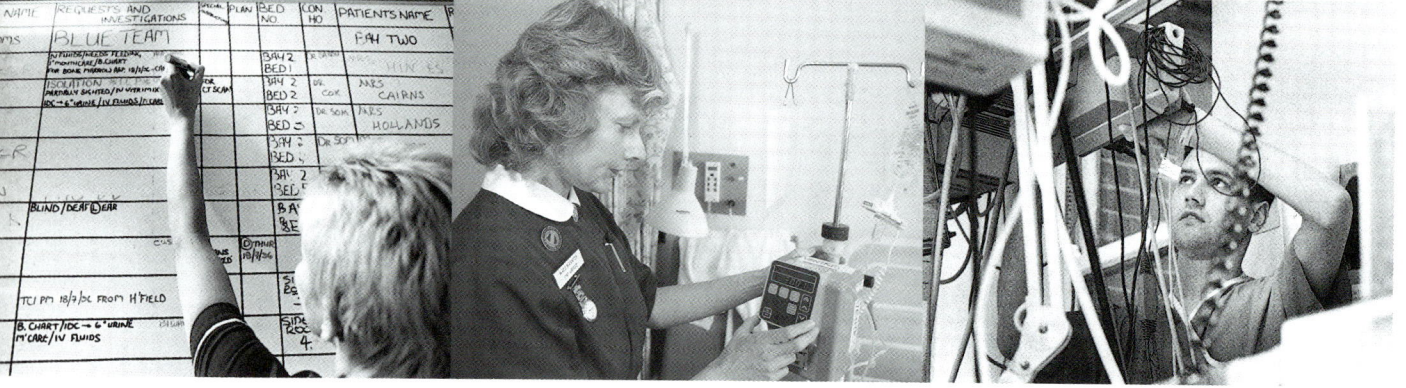

Research and the cycle of learning and practice

This Part considers some of the myths surrounding research. We help you to understand the nature of research-based knowledge and its implications for practice. We also include an introduction to evidence-based practice.

In this is included:

- A practical definition of 'research' which can help nurses understand how to be 'knowledgeable doers'

- The meaning of research-based knowledge

- Some of your strengths and weaknesses as a nurse researcher

- Some strengths and limitations of knowledge based on experience and of mutual knowledge — what 'everybody knows'

- A basic definition of evidence-based practice.

WORK PLANNER

Some of the Activities in this Section will enable you to understand research by reflecting on a topic and writing notes in your diary. However, the first Activity asks you to get together with one or two colleagues to discuss views as to how they would research a practical problem. Activity 11 also asks you to discuss a topic with your colleagues. You may want to set up both discussion topics to occur during the same period.

In the Focus Activity you are asked to keep track of various advertisements over a week. You will need to have worked through the Part before tackling the Focus Activity, but please try to leave enough time for the week it requires.

If possible, visit the Scharr Website: it supports the concepts and approaches introduced here. The address is:

http://www.shef.ac.uk/~scharr/ir/netting.html

The Further Reading list at the end of this Part suggests publications that focus on evidence-based practice.

WHAT IS RESEARCH?

Many people associate research with either classical laboratory experiments based on objectivity and fact, or theoretical research which is academic and often takes place in a university over a long period of time. However, research can also refer to the skills nurses use in their everyday practice when thinking about the most effective care to provide.

All nurses are involved in research at some stage in their professional lives. For some this might simply mean using the research skills they have developed from life in their interaction with patients and clients. These are not so different from the research skills we use when we want to find things out generally. For example, suppose you are thinking about applying for a nursing post which involves moving to another part of the country. As this is a big step which could mean a major upheaval for you and your family, you will need certain information. There are several ways you might find it:

- Talking to a colleague or friend who has lived in, or is living in, that part of the country

- Getting advice from a professional who has information about the healthcare organisation advertising the post

- Reading the organisation's annual report/national statistics

- Speaking with someone who works in the organisation already

- Driving to the area and looking around to find out what the local schools are like, the cost of housing, and so on.

ACTIVITY 1
discussion
With one or two colleagues, discuss what they would do to find out as much as they needed to know before accepting a nursing post which is far away from where they live. Would they look into all the aspects suggested above? What further details might they want to looking into and how would they go about it?

FEEDBACK

Each of the actions listed above that you might have taken, and perhaps most of those your colleagues mentioned, involve activities which are similar to the research process:

- Asking questions

- Analysing information

- Interpreting evidence

- Drawing on your own experience

- Coming to a conclusion.

At one level, then, a nurse researcher can simply refer to the ways in which information is gathered and evaluated in order to become a knowledgeable doer when interacting with patients and clients. This Part refers to research as an activity involving these kinds of skills.

ACTIVITY 2
diary
Think about a recent interaction you have had with a client which has involved any, or all, of the following activities:
• Doing a survey
• Observing and noticing things
• Reading and noting information
• Adopting a questioning approach
• Asking 'Why'; 'Is there a better way?'
Jot down in your diary which of these you do well and which you need to work on to develop. They are all important activities in research and the cycle of learning and practice in nursing.

THE VALUE OF EXPERIENCE

Utilising the skills of research gives us greater insight and knowledge about our practice. Some of these skills are used unconsciously in our everyday work. Others we are more aware of using, for instance when we read journals or articles, or talk with colleagues. Developing your research skills will help you to enhance and build on the wealth of knowledge you already possess.

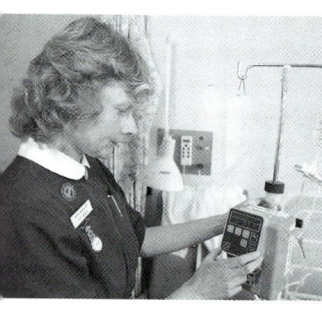

Experience is an important part of developing our knowledge base. However effective a nursing theory appears to be, if you are not able to apply it to your practice then it's not a lot of good to you. When you learn a new theory, you will need to:

• Test it out

• Analyse its effectiveness

• Think about how useful it is.

Deciding whether it is useful to you will be based on your experience of using it — the results — including what you saw, heard, felt, smelt or touched.

ACTIVITY 3
diary
Make a list of five things in your everyday life which you have learnt through your own direct experience.

Your own experience is an important element in the learning process; nothing is more vivid than seeing something for yourself rather than reading about it in a book. We can all remember 'aha' experiences, when things half-known from books suddenly become real because of our experience.

However, our own experience also has limitations.

ACTIVITY 4
diary
Think for a few moments about the sorts of experiences which you think nurses should have, with particular reference to your own nursing specialty.

The major problem with experience arises when we try to generalise from our own experience to the experience of others. For example, if you had an easy labour you might feel that someone showing a lot of signs of pain was 'making a fuss'.

However, experience can also help us to 'put ourselves in someone else's shoes'. For example, a health visitor might be more sympathetic to the problems of sleepless nights after becoming a mother herself. There have always been discussions in nursing about whether people should have had certain kinds of experiences before they come into the profession. For example:

• Should a nurse working in a hospice have experienced the death of someone else?

• Should health visitors be parents?

• Does the experience of having been nursed in bed make you a better nurse?

All these are essentially arguments about the value of personal experience.

A further problem of experience is that it is based on memories of the experience, and memory can be misleading. We do not always recall events as they really were. To illustrate this, try to remember the exact nature of your experience at breakfast this morning. What exactly happened? Of course this isn't generally a problem, but if you wanted to compare your observations of the healing of a wound six months ago, and a wound six weeks ago, do you think memory would be a good enough guide?

Notes

ACTIVITY 5
diary
How valued do you think personal knowledge is within society as a whole? Think for a moment and make some notes about the value placed on a nurse's personal experience
(a) among ordinary lay people
(b) among nurses
(c) by doctors.

FEEDBACK

Our view is that, on the whole, experience is valued more highly among lay people than among those in occupations and professions, and that nurses value it more highly than doctors. Arguments about the importance of professional learning, and of reflecting on one's own experience, are part of current thinking in nurse education. Similarly, schools now encourage pupils to value their own experience as a major source of learning.

WHAT IS RESEARCH-BASED KNOWLEDGE?

In all spheres of life we are increasingly told that new research shows that what we have been doing, with the best intentions, is wrong. For example, we are told that sugar is bad for us, that eating beef could give us 'mad cow disease', that parents should not lie babies on their tummies, or that jogging damages our joints.

You can probably think of many other examples. You may sometimes find the constant challenge to your knowledge very irritating, especially as the research seems to change and contradict itself so often. The following Activity will help you explore your own attitude to research.

ACTIVITY 6
diary
Think of one example of an area of research knowledge which you have used as the basis of a change in your life-style. Now think of an example of research which suggested that you *should* make a change in your life-style, but where you have not done so. Consider why you did not make the change. Make notes of your thoughts in your diary.

FEEDBACK

Your reason for not making a change might simply have been that you could not be bothered, but, on the other hand, you might have made a deliberate decision to reject the research. In everyday life you can choose to accept or reject research evidence, although if it turns out to be right you may have to take the consequences.

But what about using research evidence in nursing? In recent years, particularly since the Project 2000 educational reforms, the idea that nursing should be a research-based profession has become much more widely accepted, at least among the hierarchy of the profession. However, that does not mean that all nurses accept the idea — the opinions of grassroots nurses veer between wild enthusiasm and outright antagonism. Where do you come on the love/hate spectrum?

ACTIVITY 7
diary
Consider how you learnt to cook and make notes in your diary. You may have learnt from more than one source, so make notes on each of them, for example, taught by Aunt Maisie; learnt at school; still learning by experimenting and learning from mistakes; or whatever.

MUTUAL KNOWLEDGE: WHAT EVERYBODY KNOWS

Knowing what we learn from others is helpful. But the next question must be: 'Where did they get it from?'

Some of it may have come from their own experience — they are the original source of that knowledge. Sometimes this is obvious by the way they talk; they might say:

'In my experience ...'

'I have always found that ...'

'When I did ...'

'When the mountains came into view ...'

But for much of our knowledge it is not entirely clear where it comes from. Who first boiled an egg? Who decided that we would say 'Hello' when we greet someone and 'Goodbye' when we leave — and not the other way around?

Children are very good at questioning these generally known things. They ask:

'How do you know those berries are poisonous?'

'How do you know those clouds won't fall on me?'

'How do you know ladybirds don't sting?'

And the usual answer is: 'I just know ... everybody knows.'

So there is a body of knowledge which is 'what everybody knows'. This is sometimes called mutual knowledge or group knowledge. It is the knowledge that belongs to everybody in a social group. A group may be as small as a family or as large as a nation. It might be a cricket team with its mutual knowledge '... about the time when Arthur was out for a duck', or it might be inhabitants of a town who all know not to go down the High Street on a Friday evening.

It can be difficult to think consciously about this sort of knowledge. Because everybody thinks the same things we sometimes just think that's the way the world is.

'... Any member born or reared within the group accepts the ready-made standards and scheme of the cultural pattern handed down to him (or her) by ancestors, teachers, and authorities as an unquestioned and unquestionable guide in all situations which normally occur within the social world'[1].

ACTIVITY 8
diary
Can you think of two occasions when you were an outsider in a situation and realised that you didn't share the knowledge of the group? Describe them briefly in your diary.

Sociologists sometimes propose putting yourself in the position of an imaginary Martian to try and get outside your everyday perceptions of the world. They suggest you ask: How would I know what was going on in this situation? Being an outsider, although not necessarily a Martian, can help us see what everybody else takes for granted.

The Problem with Mutual Knowledge

One problem with mutual knowledge is that it is so pervasive that we hardly see it. We assume that it is what everybody knows, and anyone who doesn't know it may be labelled 'strange' or 'different'. An example of this is a comment from a ward nurse from a conventional south of England background about the problems of visiting hours. Although there was an open visiting policy for family members, she was appalled that patients who had links with other countries and cultures often had many visitors:

'Don't they know that family visiting means just one or two close family?' she bewailed.

And of course, they didn't. 'Family' in different cultures means different things. Her mutual knowledge and the patient's mutual knowledge were different and each misunderstood the other. In this case, both were right. Mutual knowledge is taken for granted between members of a group; but it must be a topic for discussion and exploration when members of two different groups meet if they are to understand each other.

So, as with our own experience, there is a limit to how far we can generalise from mutual knowledge.

Nevertheless, mutual knowledge is an enormously valuable source of information. But its use tends to be limited to dealing with current needs and circumstances, and doesn't encompass things which just might be interesting to know, but which have no apparent current use. Nor does it contain mechanisms for challenging or questioning. Belonging to a group means accepting its knowledge, not questioning it.

Questioning Mutual Knowledge

As mentioned above, those who do question mutual knowledge are likely to be considered strange or difficult, and may eventually be expelled from the group.

CASE STUDY

Margaret was a newly qualified registered nurse. Suddenly she was the senior nurse, despite the fact that there was a very experienced senior enrolled nurse in the ward, and it was expected that Margaret automatically did the office work when she was on duty. Margaret questioned whether (a) she was the more senior nurse, and (b) why the most senior nurse did the paper work and not the nursing. The night sister said that was the way things were and everybody else looked at her very strangely, so she just got on with it.

ACTIVITY 9
diary
What do you think of the justice of Margaret's case? How else do you think she could have handled it?
Can you recall an occasion when you questioned some aspect of nursing? Was it a comfortable experience? Can you describe the attitude of your colleagues?

ACTIVITY 10
diary
How far do you think the questioning of mutual knowledge is acceptable in nursing generally? What about your place of work — how much questioning goes on? Is it encouraged? Make some notes in your diary.

The questioning of mutual knowledge has led to some important changes in nursing practice, for example, whether patients need to be fasted so extensively before surgery. In midwifery, midwives began asking whether patients needed to be shaved before delivery. Why are we beginning to encourage nurses to question existing practices? Is it because change is a good thing in itself?

Why Question Mutual Knowledge?

Some of the nurses who are urging us to change might find the above questions hard to answer. One view is that there is a bit of a bandwagon in nursing, which says that change is good and staying the same is bad.

There are some much better reasons for questioning our existing practice. In our nursing practice we are trying to achieve certain things, and to achieve these things we have *choices* about how we spend the resources of time and money allocated to nursing care. This applies at all levels, from the chief executive of a trust to your own practice. You choose how to allocate the resource of your time to provide the best level of care possible in a given set of circumstances.

Being asked to make this type of choice has caused many people in the profession to question what nurses *should* be doing to make the best use of their time, and to find ways of evaluating *how well* they are doing it. We explore both these important issues in more detail in other parts of the programme.

The point to be made here is that questions such as these really concern the value of our mutual nursing knowledge.

The first of these two questions has been very much to the fore in national nursing discussions, and the issue of the mutual knowledge about what nursing is lies at the heart of it. For many years, everyone accepted that nursing, and the health service, was about dealing with what happened when people got sick. Now our mutual knowledge has changed, and we think nursing should also be concerned with preventing people getting sick. One result of this is that health promotion has become a much more prominent part of nursing than it used to be.

The second question is one which nurses 'at the coalface' are asking: *Given what we do, do we do it well enough?* And that very often leads to an exploration of the sort of knowledge we are using in practice.

Pressure to question accepted practices is also coming from outside nursing.

> **ACTIVITY 11**
> **discussion**
> Think about where the pressure to question current nursing practice is coming from outside nursing. Discuss this with one or two colleagues to find out their views.

General managers are questioning some aspects of nursing practice because they see some of it as being restrictive practice, that is, ways of working which have grown up over time but which restrict the flexibility of the workforce to respond to changing needs. Charities and pressure groups are also questioning nursing practices. For example, the National Association for the Welfare of Children in Hospital (NAWCH) questioned the practice of restricted visiting hours in children's wards, and many wards have now changed this practice, although not all.

So we can see that our mutual nursing knowledge is continually changing in response to pressures from inside and outside the profession. That it can change and adapt is one of its strengths, and one of the reasons why it remains central to nursing practice.

WHAT DO YOU CARRY INTO NURSING?

How much non-nursing knowledge do you carry into your nursing practice?

> **ACTIVITY 12**
> **diary**
> Which of these types of your personal knowledge do you use in your nursing practice?
> • Knowledge from experience
> • Mutual knowledge
> • Formal nursing knowledge.

FEEDBACK

The answer, in this case, is all of them. Essentially you are the same person at work as you are at home. You take your everyday knowledge to work with you and there you add an additional layer — your *occupational knowledge*. This does not replace your everyday knowledge but simply overlays it. It still influences the way you think and act. For instance, if, in your social group, you believe that you should be respectful to your elders, you are likely to carry this attitude into your nursing practice. If, on the other hand, your group ignores and devalues the elderly, then you are likely to see elderly people you are caring for as childlike and dependent. Of course, the converse is also true. If you learn in nursing to respect older people, you might carry that new attitude over into your everyday life.

Notes

ACTIVITY 13
diary
Think of an aspect of health, for example, headaches, periods, muscular pain, and write a statement about it which describes it in terms of:
• Your own experience
• The mutual knowledge of your group
• Formal, occupational knowledge.

FEEDBACK

Although we have spent some time looking at each of the different types of knowledge, in practice all these different strands of knowledge, both from your lay background and from your nursing knowledge, are not distinct: they are woven together, and this is why we ask you to bring your life and yourself as a person into learning. You cannot say: 'I understand that as a nurse' without being able to say 'I understand that as a person'.

AN INTRODUCTION TO EVIDENCE-BASED PRACTICE

There is more about evidence-based practice in *R2: Focusing on Research Knowledge* and *R3: Research Approaches*. In this Part, we introduce you to the basics.

You have probably heard about evidence-based practice and are perhaps already putting the principles into practice. But what is it and where did the idea come from?

The idea originated at McMaster University in Canada where practices known as 'evidence-based medicine' and 'problem-based learning' were developed. The approaches there fit in with the NHS move towards providing services, interventions and policies that are known to work.

Terms such as 'efficiency', 'effectiveness' and 'quality' are all linked to the concept of evidence-based practice. The idea is expressed by one practitioner as follows:

'Doing things cheaper + doing this better = doing things right'[2].

What is Evidence-based Practice?

Evidence-based practice is practice that has moved on from being based on intuition and experience to that based on a more informed, rational decision-making process. It has been developed after systematically reviewing current practice and new initiatives in the light of existing evidence. The rational decision-making approach concerns issues such as:

• Treatment of previously untreatable conditions

• Provision of more expensive treatments

• Increasing technology

• Treatment for individuals who would not normally receive treatment, for example those over 60; those with mental health problems, learning disabilities or severe physical disabilities; those with a gestation of under 23 weeks.

EXAMPLE

Pearce, cited in Ovretveit[3], estimated that community nurses in the UK spend 25–50% of their time treating leg ulcers, and in a study identified that nurses were not following best practice for effective treatment of leg ulcers. A profile of the nurses' caseloads, wound care costs and the number of visits made before and after implementation of evidence-based wound care was presented. The results were favourable and demonstrated a reduction in expenditure on wound care products, a saving in nurses' time and a reduction in caseload numbers.

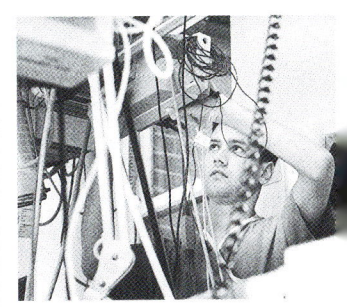

Notes

A Continuous Treatment Process

Evidence-based practice concerns clinical effectiveness and is a continuous process:

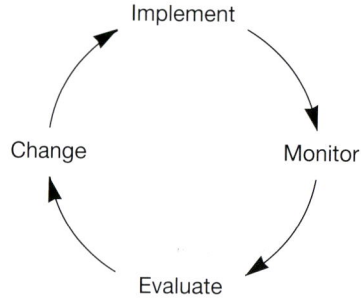

Like all good practice in nursing, evidence-based practice should be seen and used as an important tool. But it does not discount the value of nurses' own experience or of mutual knowledge[2-4].

FOCUS

During the next week keep a close check on the ways in which advertisements appeal to the different types of knowledge: scientific knowledge — 'scientifically proven to ...'; mutual knowledge — 'everybody agrees that'; and experiential knowledge — 'try it and see for yourself'. Make notes in your diary of advertisements on TV and radio. Advertisements in papers and journals can be cut out and put in your files.

See if there is any difference between advertisements directed at you as an ordinary person and you as a nurse.

REFERENCES

1 Schutz, A. The stranger: An essay in social psychology. In: Brodesen, A. (ed) *Studies in Social Theory (Collected Papers II)*. The Hague: Martinus Nijhoff, 1964.
2 Muir, Gray, J.A. *Evidence-based Healthcare*. London: Churchill Livingstone, 1997.
3 Ovretveit, J. *Evaluating Health Interventions*. Buckingham: Open University Press, 1998.
4 Jenkinson, C. *Assessment and Evaluation in Health Care*. Buckingham: Open University Press, 1998.

FURTHER READING

• Jack, B., Oldham, J. Taking steps towards evidence-based practice: A model for implementation. *Nurse Researcher* 1997; **5**: 1, 65–71.
• McClarey, M. Clinical effectiveness and evidence-based practice. *Nursing Standard* 1997; **11**: 52, 33–37.
• Robinson, D., Gajos, M., Whyte, L. Integrating research into practice: A model for evidence-based care through ward-based learning. *Psychiatric Care* 1997; **4**: 6, 274–278.

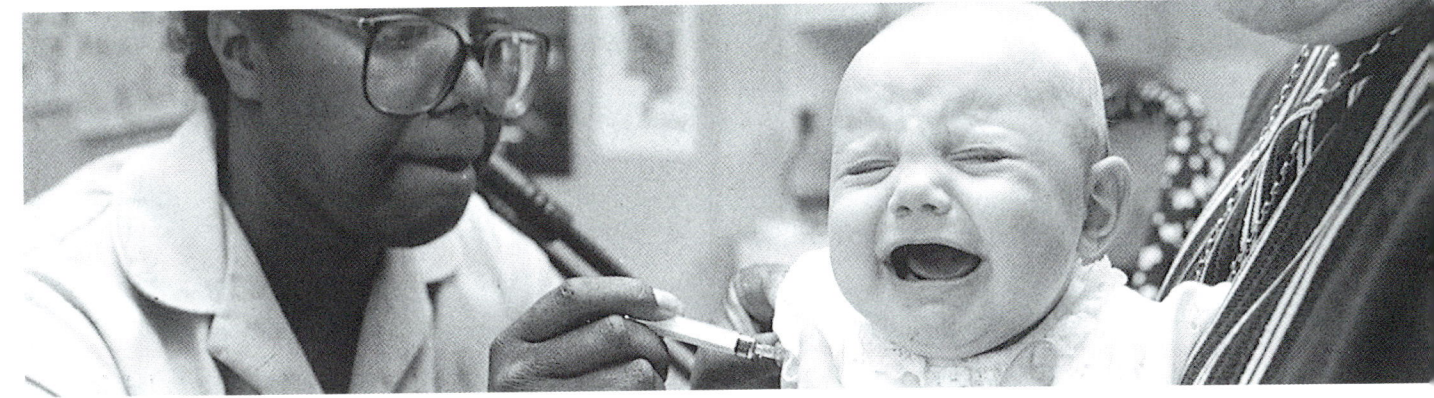

A personal view of health and illness

Notes

Does everyone share the same ideas of health and illness? In this first Part of *Health and Illness* you consider:

- A definition of good health
- Different attitudes to health and how age, gender and social class influence attitudes
- How we decide whether we are ill and how we feel about taking time off work owing to illness
- How you maintain good health for yourself.

WORK PLANNER

The Focus Activity for this Part asks you to carry out a mini-survey to find out more about factors which affect people's ideas of health and illness.

You will need to identify two people, one male and one female if possible, from each decade of life (that is, under 10, 11-20, 21-30 and so on) up to 90+ if possible. You will probably find that you interview between 15 and 20 people.

As with any interview you carry out as part of your work on this programme, you should prepare what you are going to say in advance. When you ask the person's permission to carry out the interview, explain the purpose of the interview and emphasise that it will be treated as confidential. You will find more guidance on preparing for interviews in your student pack.

GOOD HEALTH

Begin by thinking about your own health.

ACTIVITY 1
diary
Describe your present state of health, using as few words as possible. Then describe your most recent illness, explaining:
- What it was
- How you decided you were ill.

FEEDBACK

To have made any judgement about your present state of health, you must have used some idea of 'good health' or 'ill health' against which to measure it.

ACTIVITY 2
diary
Write a definition of good health that could be applied to anyone in the world.

FEEDBACK

The World Health Organization (WHO) is an international organisation concerned with making a positive contribution to the health of all those who live on this planet. The WHO defines health as:

'A state of complete physical, mental and social well-being and not merely the absence of disease or infirmity'[1].

Did your definition include all three aspects of well-being:

- Physical

- Mental

- Social?

Social Well-being

Because human beings rarely live in complete isolation from one another, the conduct of each individual affects others. If you have ever lived next door to a noisy neighbour, you may have felt your social well-being severely threatened.

Social well-being and health are very closely related and any view of health that excludes the social setting in which an individual lives is not a complete one. It is fairly easy to see how factors such as damp living conditions, inadequate clothing and even noise can lead to ill health, but social pressures can have equally devastating effects.

CASE STUDY

Hari was a student nurse. He came to England from Asia with his family when he was a baby and grew up with a wide range of friends of many different ethnic, cultural and religious backgrounds. When he was 19 Hari acknowledged to himself that he was gay but none of his family or the friends who had contact with them were aware of it. Six months before completion of his training, Hari's father told him that arrangements had been made for him to return to the country in which he had been born for an arranged marriage. The wedding had been planned to take place during his next holiday in three months' time. Hari became very distressed but felt that he could not reveal his complex problems to anyone. He lost a great deal of weight, was unable to concentrate at work and repeatedly suffered from streaming colds. The week before his holiday, Hari failed to report on duty. When his nursing manager contacted his parents she was told that he had left a note saying that he had gone away.

Three weeks later, Hari arrived at the home of one of his fellow students and told her the whole story, including the fact that he had spent the past three weeks living rough. He was desperately depressed and had constantly thought of suicide but believed that he had the right to live his life as he wanted and not as his family and culture dictated.

ACTIVITY 3
diary
Can you think of anyone whose health has been affected by his/her social situation? Describe the person's health and the reasons behind your thoughts.

ATTITUDES TO HEALTH

Notes

Most of our opinions about the way we feel about health and illness result from the experiences to which we have been exposed and the opinions we have heard from other people. These may go back to our childhood: how we were treated by parents and grandparents when we were hurt or unwell. This idea is supported by research. Fitzpatrick[2] describes the way people experience illness as being influenced by the culture of the society in which they live. So a person's reaction to illness and the action he or she takes is the result of the accepted ways of behaving within the social group of which that person is a part.

Self-Concept

Because we make personal judgements about our own state of health, it follows that our health is a vital part of the way in which we see ourselves – our 'self-concept'. Baxter and Paterson[3] sum it up by pointing out that we live in our bodies and that our physical identity is part of ourselves.

CASE STUDY

Albert is 81. He grew up in a large family which experienced much hardship. He describes himself as having been an athlete in his youth. He now has severe arterial insuffiency in his legs, which is impossible to correct surgically. He has a severe flexion contracture in one knee and can only just put the foot to the ground to enable him to hobble from bed to chair. Going for any sort of outing or even in the garden is virtually impossible. The pain from his legs is so severe that Albert never gets more than a few hours sleep at a time, having to take analgesia during the night when the pain wakes him. During the day he catnaps to catch up on his sleep. Despite all this, Albert will not countenance an amputation, even though it would give a strong chance of restoring a degree of mobility. He will not consider the possibility because he sees amputees as 'cripples'. Physical fitness was everything to Albert as a young man.

ACTIVITY 4
diary
Do you know people – friends, family, clients, patients – in whom you can identify cultural or social aspects of their lives which have influenced the way they think about their health? Write a brief description of each one.
Are these influences positive, or negative, as in Albert's case?

Stigmatisation

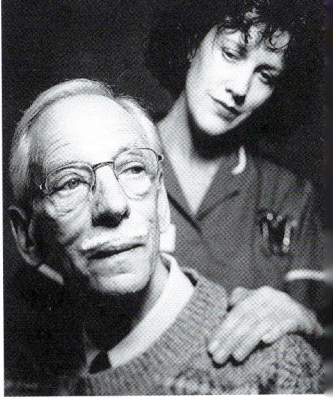

The idea of illness causing an individual to be held in low regard by others is often referred to as 'stigmatisation'. A wide range of illnesses, such as AIDS, psoriasis, diabetes and deafness has been shown to be stigmatising[4]. Such stigmatisation may be something people feel within themselves or it may be that they experience negative attitudes from other people as well. Albert felt that amputation was stigmatising, the low regard coming from his own feelings, although they resulted from his early years. If he had undergone an amputaion and experienced contempt or, more subtly, loss of status as a result, he would have been stigmatised by others. The degree to which illnesses are stigmatised varies, and mental disability is usually a greater stigma than physical illness[5].

ACTIVITY 5
diary
What illnesses or health problems would you personally feel stigmatised by if you had them?

Different Groups

Within any culture there are different groups. This section looks at:

- Age

- Gender

- Social class.

Age

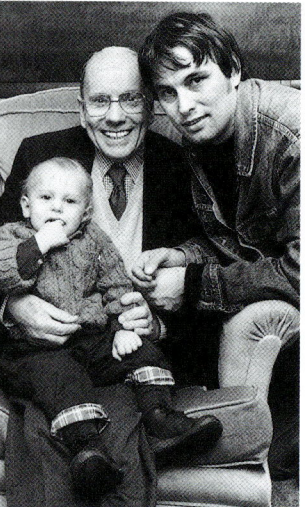

Does age make a difference? A study by Williams[6] indicated that it does. His study particularly noted that the over-sixties saw health as the absence of disease, which is a relatively neutral state lacking any positive claims to health.

You may say that this is only to be expected because as people get older they would tend to be realistic about the degree of health they could expect to enjoy. That is probably true, but is not invariably so.

ACTIVITY 6
diary
What differences due to age have you noticed among young people you know in their attitude to health? Make some notes. Have you come across any younger people who have a more limited view of health expectations than older people? Or the other way round? Make a note of the reasons for this.

Gender

Does gender affect our attitudes to health? Are there differences between men and women in ideas of what health is? This is more difficult to answer, but there is evidence that the idea of health as 'positive fitness' is seen more often in men than in women[7].

A possible controversial explanation for this is that from puberty women experience menstruation, which is often accompanied by pain, nausea and other problems. Then, as many women experience pregnancy, childbirth and lactation, they feel that good health is being free from discomfort rather than a positive state of feeling healthy.

Social class

Social class may also have a bearing on views of health and illness. Just as increasing age tends to lower expectations of health, so membership of a lower social class appears to produce a similar, and probably realistic, outlook. A study by Pill and Stott[8] of working-class mothers revealed that they had a broad view of health in that they regarded it as the 'absence of illness', which lacked any positive aspect such as 'feeling full of energy' or 'being really fit'.

ACTIVITY 7
diary
Think about one or both of your parents and their social backgrounds. Can you see any difference between their health expectations when you were a child and your own now? Make a note of any you can identify.

The evidence from research seems to be that we should never take our own viewpoint or definition of health as being the same as that of any other person, whether family, friend or patient.

ATTITUDES TO ILLNESS

In Activity 1 you described your most recent illness. It is important to think carefully about what led you to believe you were ill. The things you used to describe that you were ill will be an indication of what you think illness is. There are some serious implications here, because the 'rules' we use to decide if we are ill may affect the number and types of illnesses from which we suffer.

ACTIVITY 8
diary
Look back to your answer to Activity 1 and your description of your most recent illness. If at that or some other time you had to report sick because you were so ill that you could not go into work, you must have had to give some explanation to your manager. Think back to the last occasion on which that happened and describe, as closely as possible, how you described your illness and the reasons you gave for being unable to work.

FEEDBACK

Cornwell[9] concluded that there seems to be a moral aspect to the subject of illness. She found during her research that if people had mentioned illness, they took care to ensure that it was understood that they were real illnesses. There may be an underlying belief in many people that illness must be diagnostically proved.

Do you feel an obligation to prove your illness when you are absent from work?

Personal Responsibility

This sort of feeling ties in with evidence that individuals feel a responsibilty for their health and for anything that detracts from it[10]. This may not be a logical attitude since we cannot avoid exposure to infectious organisms such as influenza or cold viruses if we mix with other people at all.

ACTIVITY 9
diary
Have another look at your 'reporting sick' explanation from Activity 8. Consider and note down how far you felt it necessary to prove your illness.

We may feel guilty at becoming ill because we feel we have let down family or colleagues. Group differences may play a part in feelings about illness, as they do in ideas about health.

ACTIVITY 10
diary
Do you think there are any differences between the way men as opposed to women feel able to declare themselves 'sick' and stop working? You may have experiences of your own which show the differences.

Cornwell, in the article referred to above, found that men and women had very different responses to feeling unwell and this was seen as being closely related to how easy it was for the sick person to avoid work. Paid employment, more usually the major employment of men, is often more avoidable than the constant demands made on a wife and mother who is frequently expected to take total responsibility for feeding and caring for a family. (In a household in which domestic labour is not decided on a gender basis this would obviously not apply.)

STAYING WELL

ACTIVITY 11
diary
Do you feel that you have a personal responsibility to take positive steps to reach and maintain a good level of health? Describe in a few sentences the reasons for your answer.

FEEDBACK

You may have found yourself coming back to some of the factors already considered when talking about becoming ill, such as feeling a moral responsibility for your own health, or your obligations to other people such as family and work colleagues.

Notes

ACTIVITY 12
diary
Describe the action you take at present to ensure your own good health.

FEEDBACK

How did you decide on the action you are taking, or not taking as the case may be? Did you just drift into something like a high-fibre diet because your partner stocks the food cupboard and prefers high-fibre items, or did you see a stunning newspaper headline promising an early grave if you didn't mend your ways? Did you perhaps go out and read all the research literature on the subject of a healthy life-style before deciding to embrace or reject part or all of the researched-based recommendations?

Even if you are well informed and have made a logical decision actively to build up your own health levels, you may find that other factors have to be considered, such as time, money and even the energy necessary to change to healthier habits!

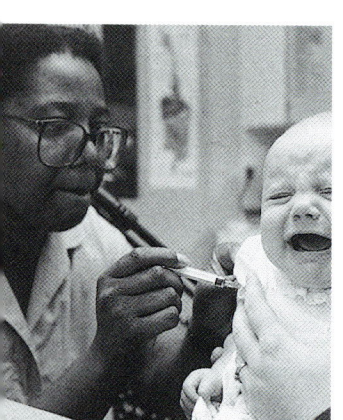

This business of deciding what health and illness are, or what they mean to different people, and what action an individual should or might take to promote good health, is very complicated! It is even more complicated for us as a group because, as well as being the individuals known to our family and friends, we are also nurses, whose responsibilities include health education generally and helping individual patients to recover and maintain the highest level of health possible for them.

'Health nursing is … the process of promoting health through nursing care. … Health nursing will not be achieved until the philosophy underpinning practice is grounded in the principles of enhancing health. A rejection of sick nursing is required in order that the internalised goals of nursing become linked to the promotion of health. Such a rejection must surely constitute a professional revolution[11].'

You might be interested to read *Health Promotion in Professional Practice*[12] which goes into these issues further.

One major problem is that there is conflicting information coming from a wide variety of groups with input into healthcare. The remaining parts in this Section, *P1(ii): Health and power* and *P1(iii): Professionals and consumers* look at how different groups have contributed to ideas on health and illness and the consequences of particular definitions of them to nursing practice.

FOCUS

Before starting work on this Activity, read the notes in the Work Planner for this Part.

Ask the following questions of each person you have identified:

- 'What is your definition of health?'

- 'Can you remember the last time you had a minor illness?' (cold, flu, or suggest other appropriate examples)

- 'How did you feel about the illness, and why do you think you felt this way?'

When you have completed the interviews (which should take about 10 minutes each), prepare a report (no more than two pages) of your findings about how age and gender affect people's views on health and illness. Depending on who your interviewees were, you may also be able to add some findings on the influence of other factors, such as social class or ethnic background.

You may wish to negotiate with your tutor and student group to deliver your report to them orally during a group study session, rather than as a piece of written work.

REFERENCES

1   Hogarth, J. *Glossary of Healthcare Terminology. Public health in Europe Number 4.* Copenhagen:WHO Regional Office for Europe, 1975.

2   Fitzpatrick, R. Lay concepts of illness. In: Fitzpatrick R., Hinton J., Newman S., Thompson J. *The Experience of Illness.* London: Tavistock Publications, 1984.

3   Baxter, M., Paterson L. The cause of disease: Women talking. *Social Science and Medicine* 1982; **17**: 2, 59–69.

4   Scambler, G. Perceiving and coping with stigmatising illness. In: Fitzpatrick R., Hinton J., Newman S., Thompson J. *The Experience of Illness.* London: Tavistock Publications, 1984.

5   Furnham, A., Pendred J. Attitudes towards the mentally and physically disabled. *British Journal of Medical Psychology* 1983; **56**: 179–187.

6   Williams, R. Concepts of health: An analysis of lay logic. *Sociology* 1983; **17**: 185–204.

7   Stacey, M. *The Sociology of Health and Healing.* London: Unwin Hyman Ltd, 1988.

8   Pill, R. Stott, N. Concepts of illness causation and responsibility: Some preliminary data from a sample of working class mothers. *Social Science and Medicine* 1982; **16**: 1, 43–52.

9   Cornwell, J. *Hard-earned lives. Accounts of health and illness from East London.* Tavistock Publications, 1984.

10 Herzlich, C. *Health and Illness.* London: Academic Press, 1973.

11 Macleod Clarke, J. From sick nursing to health nursing: Evolution or revolution? In: Wilson-Barnett, J., Macleod Clarke, J. (eds). *Research in Health Promotion and Nursing.* Basingstoke: Macmillan Press, 1993.

12 Macmillan Open Learning [Emap Healthcare Open Learning]. *Health Promotion in Professional Practice.* London: Macmillan Magazines Ltd, 1997.

Notes

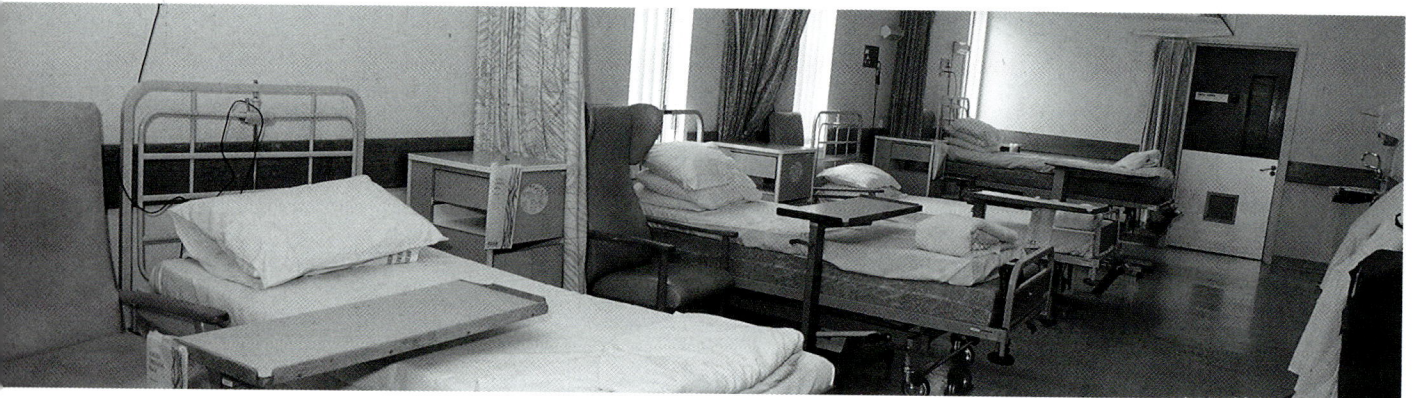

Notes

Health and power

This Part of *Health and Illness* considers the influence of various power groups on our ideas of health and illness. These groups come under four headings:

- Political
- Professional
- Economic
- Representational.

The key points in this Part include:

- Financing healthcare: individuals or state?
- Health as a political decision
- The role of doctors in influencing our attitudes on health
- The power of drug companies.

WORK PLANNER

You will need a copy of *The Patient's Charter* for Activity 4.

You will also need to schedule time for Activity 5, which is a discussion topic. You will need to approach two or three colleagues to take part in this Activity with you.

HEALTH FOR ALL?

Part (i): A personal view of health and illness asked you to think about the different ways in which we as individuals view health and illness. In this Part (P1: (ii)) we consider how various groups in society influence our attitudes, and the power they have to determine the provision of healthcare.

Think about the factors which influence good health.

In 1978 the WHO issued a challenge to the world to attain health for all by the year 2000, and subsequently, in 1986[1] their European office defined 38 health targets, summarised below.

WHO Health Targets

The pre-requisites for health

- Peace
- Social justice
- Adequate and wholesome food
- Safe water
- Decent housing and sanitation for everyone
- Education for everyone
- Secure employment so that everyone has a valued and rewarding role in society.

The targets

Equity in health so that everyone has the best possible opportunity to develop healthily and to obtain the required healthcare

The addition to years of life by the prevention of premature death

The addition of health to life so that preventable disease and disability are minimised

The addition of life to years so that the highest attainable level of health continues to be enjoyed by both the elderly and those disabled by chronic illness or permanent impairment

Identification and promotion of healthy behaviour and the discouragement of unhealthy behaviour

The introduction of policies in all sectors of public life to make it easier to adopt healthy life-styles and to participate in health policy-making; and to enhance the family or other social groupings

The creation and preservation of a **healthy environment**

The development of health services which are appropriate to people's needs and wishes

Acceptance of these goals by those responsible for research, for service management and for training within the health professions.

The action needed to achieve targets such as these on a large scale can be taken only by groups of people with enough power in society to carry them through.

In a developed Western country, a majority of people could take for granted most of the pre-requisites for health. The situation in a less developed country can be quite different.

**ACTIVITY 1
knowledge base**
Think about a less developed country where many of the pre-requisites for health are not in place. What groups in that society do you think could have the power to ensure that the WHO health targets are met? Suggest one or two reasons why these targets have not been achieved before now.

FEEDBACK
Some of the groups you may have thought of are: governments, healthcare workers, teachers and charities. Key reasons why such groups are often unable to achieve very much are political instability and war.

Notes

GROUPS WITH POWER

In a democracy, individuals are able to form groups to put across a particular message and to campaign for changes. These groups can have a lot of power. Some groups use the media to increase awareness and gain support, for example, campaigns by trade unions. Other groups may take legal or illegal actions to raise awareness, for example, animal welfare groups.

There are groups in our society which hold the power to influence people's idea of health and illness.

ACTIVITY 2
discussion
Can you think of some of the groups which influence our society on health matters?

FEEDBACK

Some groups you may have noted down are the Health Education Council, big charities such as the British Heart Foundation which puts across a strong message on how to avoid heart disease, or groups campaigning for safe sex.

ACTIVITY 3
action
Over the next few days, pick up leaflets from charities or organisations dealing with health matters. Look at any health messages they are putting across and think about how effective they are.

FEEDBACK

What factors give a group power? Your list might include: already holding power, having money, having knowledge, having some means of making views public. We can group these factors under four headings:

- Political
- Professional
- Economic
- Representational.

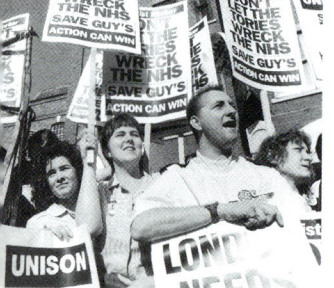

POLITICAL POWER

Any political group in power, even in a democracy which has voted it into government, exerts a tremendous influence on perceptions of health. The National Health Service was a dream realised by those whose political beliefs focused on the right of everyone in society to free social welfare and healthcare. It was set up to ensure that everyone in Britain had equal access to healthcare, regardless of his or her personal financial circumstances.

Unlimited funds?

Any government can spend only the money it has available. To have more money available it will have to increase taxation. Overall, however much money a government has, it will have to make decisions on what proportion of that money goes to education, to health, to defence, and so on.

The White Paper, *The New NHS: Modern, dependable*[2], has this to say:

> The Government is committed to the historic principle that if you are ill or injured there will be a national health service to help; and access to it will be based on need and need alone – not on your ability to pay or on who your GP happens to be or where you live. The *New NHS* sets out how the internal market will be replaced by a system of integrated care, based on partnership and driven by performance. Abolishing the internal market will cut £1 billion of red tape costs over the lifetime of the Parliament for investment in patient care.

As we have already seen, the decision as to what a country can afford to spend on health, as opposed to transport or any other sort of government spending, is a political decision. Cervical smears or six-lane motorways? If a choice of the latter means that we can't 'afford' the technicians necessary to scan smears adequately, leading to a reduction in the number that can be done, our perception of health as a positive state may be reduced.

EXAMPLE

There have already been situations where transplant surgery has been limited by shortage of funds to pay for it. Techniques are now developing very rapidly indeed and success levels rising. We may soon reach a situation where, technically, there are no reasons for limiting such major surgery. Where will the money come from to pay for it? It is likely that medical advances will outstrip the money available, even if there were a high level of taxation and the income was spent on very little else but healthcare.

The Patient's Charter

In 1991, in an attempt to answer criticism that its policies would lead to a reduction in the amount and quality of state-funded healthcare in the United Kingdom, the government published *The Patient's Charter*[3]. This set out what the government saw as the basic healthcare rights of every individual, and is therefore a statement by one group with power about what healthcare should be.

ACTIVITY 4
Knowledge base
1. Read *The Patient's Charter*, and make some notes about what you think were the priorities of those who wrote it. How feasible do you think it is in your area of practice to ensure that these rights are met for every client?
2. Find out about *Fairness at Work*[4], a White Paper published in 1998 by the Department of Trade and Industry. It deals with the way in which employees – individually or collectively – and their employers interact. Do you see any conflict between the requirements placed upon you as a nurse under *The Patient's Charter* and the requirements of employees as set out in *Fairness at Work*?

Owen[5] pointed out that public opinion does not always choose the same priorities as do those in government and management, whose job it is to plan the health service.

How much healthcare should people be entitled to? There is an enormous range of possibilities. Britain in the past had a system by which very little healthcare at all was available unless the patient was able to pay as and when help was required. Many countries use this model of healthcare.

Equally, it is theoretically possible to give full healthcare to everyone without payment being made at the time of use, starting with health promotion before conception, including child healthcare with subsidised nutrition in the form of school milk and meals, medical consultation and treatment, and social support available on request and without means testing.

ACTIVITY 5
discussion
In an ideal world, what sort of healthcare provision do you think would be best for everyone in our society? Would you go for all care paid for by individuals as they need it, all paid for by the state from money raised from everyone in society, or some mixture of the two? Discuss these issues with colleagues and give reasons for the choice you make.

FEEDBACK

Whether healthcare is a personal or national responsibility, there is one basic truth: we can still only spend what we can afford. How can this be achieved? If you believe that we should all pay for our own healthcare, the answer is that each individual must insure against illness or save enough to be able to pay any bills for healthcare. In such a system anyone who cannot pay the insurance premiums or the bills will either rely on charity or go without healthcare.

Choices

The outcome of these issues is that choices will have to be made about what is a 'reasonable' level of health care and what is not. These sorts of choices are already being made in a limited way by healthcare professionals, health authorities, health department officials and politicians. Where is the cut-off point for providing state-funded healthcare for all members of society?

One way in which the 1997 White Paper, *The New NHS: Modern, dependable*[2], aims to cut costs and promote more efficient and effective use of resources is by capping management costs. How will this affect the environment in which you are working?

Whatever personal choice you made in Activity 5 for funding healthcare, you may already be faced with choices being made in allocating resources in your own nursing sphere. When you are a qualified nurse you may be involved in the process of deciding what care it is reasonable to expect the state to fund and which conditions, or groups of patients, will be excluded.

ACTIVITY 6
discussion
Think about your own specialty. You are told that savings have to be made. Can you identify any resources and/or aspects of care for which a client could reasonably be expected to pay?

FEEDBACK

You may find this a difficult question to answer. Many others have also found this to be the case. It is the question at the heart of the current political debate about the future of the NHS. The way that those with political power answer this question will determine the way healthcare is provided in the years to come.

PROFESSIONAL POWER

We have said that in the British system, healthcare is intended to be available to anyone who needs it, but here we run into further problems because it is professional experts in healthcare who define and identify what is need[6].

The following paragraphs explore the influence and power that the medical profession has on people's views of health and illness.

The Biomedical Model

You may have heard the term 'biomedical model' used when health and illness are described. It means that when health and illness are considered, any disease can be fully accounted for by medical factors, such as measurable differences in normal body functions.

ACTIVITY 7
knowledge base
Think of half-a-dozen health/illness conditions that can be measured in this way; hypertension or ulcerative colitis are two examples. Can you think of two problems which arise when using this model?

FEEDBACK

There are two basic problems in using this model as a means of identifying need in healthcare. The first problem is that although there is a range of biochemical factors that do have normal upper and lower limits, such as blood potassium levels, there are many factors whose 'normality' can be hotly debated; for example, what is a 'normal' night's sleep?

The second problem with this model is that it suggests that if what you feel is wrong with you cannot be measured, because there is no test for it, it doesn't exist. You therefore haven't got it, and you are, by implication, not ill! Sufferers from myalgic encephalomyelitis (ME) have experienced this problem. The biomedical model also ignores social, psychological and other aspects of illness.[7]

The Doctor's Influence

One of the most powerful influences on our attitudes to health and illness is what our doctors say to us. Doctors have knowledge and experience on health matters which most people do not have. Traditionally, doctors have been held in awe by many members of society, and today even if we don't hold quite those views, we rely heavily on them to enable us to overcome ill health.

ACTIVITY 8
discussion

Do you think doctors are always the most appropriate professional group to influence the public's attitudes to health? What other professionals could have a role? For example, many expectant mothers find that the advice they get from their midwives is more helpful than information from their doctors.

ECONOMIC POWER

There are a number of economic power groups whose activities may affect our ideas of health and illness. These include those who provide private healthcare and those whose products are used in both the private and state sectors.

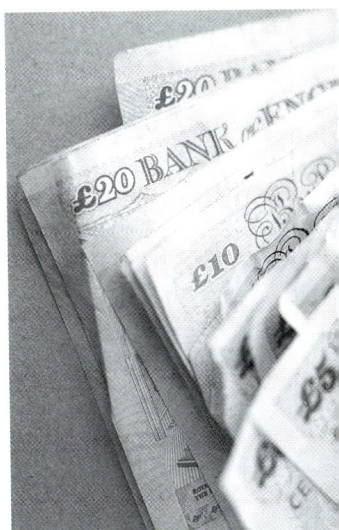

EXAMPLE

Several decades ago the idea of having a breast reduction was virtually unknown among the general population, and many women suffered great discomfort. While breast reduction was possible within the state system, it was limited to a very small number of women and consequently there was very little public awareness. It is only since increased private healthcare has enabled more women to undergo this surgery that its benefits have become widely known and more women have requested help from the state sector.

EXAMPLE

Drugs are another example where financial considerations have affected public perceptions of healthcare, this time not just in knowing that they are available but in making choices between them and other forms of treatment. It is hard these days to imagine nursing without drugs, because they have become a mainstay of healthcare. This was not always so, and indeed it is only in the past 20 years that we have had so many drugs with which to treat illness.

Where does the money come from to develop new drugs? Some of it is given in the form of research grants, often from charitable foundations, but much of it is provided by drug firms themselves who plough back profits from drugs they are already producing. The uptake of existing products is therefore an important factor in future development.

Increasingly we live in a consumer culture. When we shop for clothes or food most of us have expectations about the quality of our purchase. So, for example, food manufacturers are required to label the content and sell-by date of each product. We also, in turn, have expectations about the quality and service of the healthcare provided. The number of complaints made to trusts is rising, and the nature of the complaints is increasingly complex as we challenge all aspects of care received. NHS trusts are also required to cut their waiting lists, and a new system of clinical governance has been introduced to ensure that clinical standards are met and that there are processes to ensure continuous improvement. There is now a statutory duty for quality in all NHS trusts.

REPRESENTATIONAL POWER

Political power, professional power and economic power all contribute to what society generally, and each of us as individuals, sees as 'health' or as 'illness'. The influence of each of these groups helps subconsciously, and often consciously, to form our values and therefore to affect the demands we make for healthcare.

Notes

There is one further type of power group which we listed at the start of this unit: groups of people who join together specifically to represent a certain point of view, or the needs of a particular group. Such consumer groups can play an important role in healthcare, and have a particular significance for us as nurses.

ACTIVITY 9
diary
Before you tackle the Focus, identify one or more ways in which the four power groups you have looked at have made an impact on your area of professional practice.

As nurses we are in a position to exert influence ourselves, both as a professional group and as individuals. As consumers of healthcare we may feel as helpless and powerless as anyone else. The Community Health Council (CHC) has a powerful role to play in supporting and reflecting the views of local people about their health service. The particular definitions that nurses have of health and illness can have very far-reaching consequences for nursing practice, and in *P1(iii): Professionals and consumers*, our final look for the time being at health and illness, we turn the spotlight on nursing and the consumer.

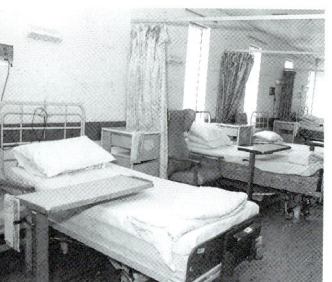

FOCUS

1. Choose one of the power groups which has influenced or will influence the provision of care in your specialist area.

2. Write a short report (about one side of A4) summarising:

   A. What this group has done or said to influence the way care is or will be provided

   B. How any resulting changes have come about — were they imposed, or did they evolve?

REFERENCES

1   World Health Organization. *Health for All by the Year 2000. Charter for action.* London: The Faculty of Community Medicine, 1986.

2   Department of Health. *The New NHS: Modern, dependable.* London: The Stationery Office, Cmnd 3807, 1997.

3   Department of Health. *The Patient's Charter.* London: HMSO, 1991.

4   Department of Trade and Industry. *Fairness at Work.* (White Paper). London: Department of Trade and Industry, 1998.

5   Owen, D. *In Sickness and in Health.* London: Quartet Books Ltd, 1976.

6   Klein, R. The politics of participation. In: Maxwell, R., Weaver, N. (eds). *Public Participation in Health.* London: King Edward's Hospital Fund, 1984.

7   Engel, G.L. The need for a new medical model: A challenge for bio-medicine. *Science* 1977; **196**: 4286, 120–136.

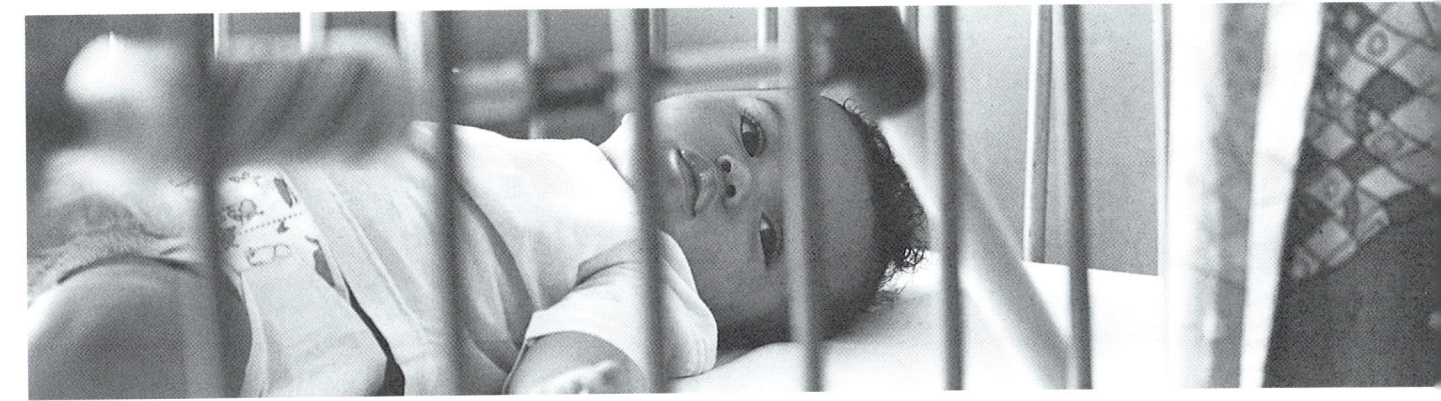

Professionals and consumers

How do you know what consumers of healthcare want? This Part looks at:

- The dangers of professional health carers exploiting their status
- Different groups which represent consumers of healthcare
    - community health councils
    - self-help groups
- Ways in which you can learn from self-help groups and enrich your nursing practice.

WORK PLANNER

For Activity 3 you will need to get a copy of the last annual report of your health council.

Make sure you have your copy of *The Patient's Charter* which you may have looked at in *P1(ii): Health and power*. You will need this for Activity 4.

For Activity 6 a useful directory is *The Voluntary Agencies Directory* (published by NCVO Publishers (1998)). You will also need a list of local self-help groups, which you can find in your local library or from your local Council for Voluntary Service.

We suggest some discussion in Activities 4, 5 and 8, so you will need to allocate some time for this.

HEALTHCARE PROFESSIONALS

P1(i): A personal view of health and illness looked at different ideas people have about health and illness, and *P1(ii): Health and power* considered healthcare power groups. This Part looks at the role of professionals in more detail. Healthcare is often seen as a 'them and us' situation — 'we' the professionals, and 'them', the general public, often referred to as the lay public or the laity. How these two 'sides' view each other is of crucial importance in determining the type of healthcare that is available. Do healthcare professionals cling to their special knowledge, and use it to keep the consumer, and consumer opinion, at bay?

Notes

ACTIVITY 1
diary
What is your opinion about the way in which healthcare professionals guard their position? Choose from the statements alongside the one you most agree with as a healthcare professional. Make a note in your diary.

In my experience, healthcare professionals generally:

(a) Tell people what care/treatment they need with little or no discussion

(b) Give the impression of discussing needs but still actually define and decide them for clients

(c) Undertake full and open discussion while giving professional advice, without waiting to be asked

(d) Discuss known facts and give a professional opinion when specifically asked.

Which of these approaches do you think clients generally would prefer, and why?

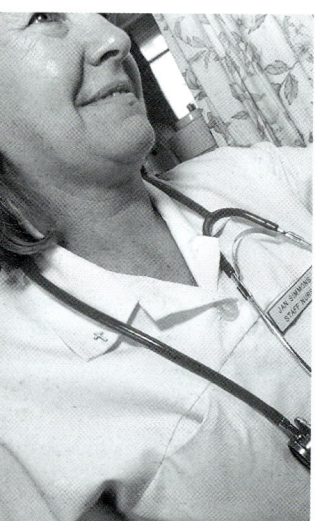

Does Nurse Know Best?

Do nurses as healthcare professionals have the right to believe that they may know better than other members of society what other people's healthcare needs are? Clearly, our training and experience give us the authority to make the sort of judgement that results from a nursing process evaluation of specific nursing needs, such as the particular care a person with plaster of Paris splintage requires. But is this true at a more general level?

As people who watch television, read newspapers and even the relevant research reports, we are entitled to have an opinion on this particular subject or indeed on any other subject. However, problems may arise if we use our professional status to give our personal opinions extra weight or credibility.

EXAMPLE

An off-duty nurse is having lunch with friends. She makes the remark: 'Well, as a nurse, I think that irradiating food is a terrible risk.'

There are great dangers in making comments like this. This nurse believes that her opinion is more valid because she is a nurse. By making the statement she may also have influenced what her friends think about irradiation of food. In other words, her use of her professional status may affect other people's perceptions of health and health risks.

The example underlines the strong argument that professionals have become exclusive experts on the public good[1]. While it would be stupid to deny that professionals have expertise, it is the belief that only professionals have valid opinions or that as professionals their opinions always carry more weight than others, that is the danger.

ACTIVITY 2
diary
For your diary's eyes only, consider if, on reflection, you have ever used your professional status to give weight to your beliefs in a general discussion. What were the circumstances? Can you work out exactly why you did it and why you felt at the time that it was the right thing to do? Do you still think it was the right thing to have done?

Now we look at different groups which represent consumers of healthcare. You will consider whether you can take action on anything you learn from consumer groups.

THE CONSUMER FIGHTS BACK

Whenever we talk about health we must talk about society, because it is people who are considered to be healthy or not, and it is people who are society[2].

As explained in *P1(i): A personal view of health and illness*, ideas of what health is are rooted in the society in which we live. There are a number of statutory and voluntary bodies through which consumers can make their views known. Such groups make it possible for those not in powerful positions to make their voices heard.

Community Health Councils

A statutory body is a group whose existence is enforced by law. Until 1974 there had never been a completely separate body to represent the public's view of health care. In 1973, however, the NHS Reorganisation Act gave the secretary of state the duty to establish community health councils (CHCs) or, in Scotland, local health councils (LHCs). In Northern Ireland, the equivalent district committees were replaced in 1990 by area health and social services councils.

All these councils are similarly structured. They have a variety of members, a proportion of whom must be appointed by the local authorities and by voluntary organisations. The remainder must be appointed after consultation with the local authorities and the other bodies the regional health authority (RHA) considers appropriate. Each health council must produce an annual report to the RHA and also make that report public.

ACTIVITY 3
action
Get hold of the last annual report of your local health council or community health council and take a critical look at the list of health council members. Are they a representative cross-section of your community? Which organisations are represented? Do you think there is an equal balance between men and women, and different age, cultural and ethnic groups? You will need the report again for the next Activity.

FEEDBACK

The regulations state that each council should keep under review the operation of health services in its district and make recommendations for improvement. Although each CHC may approach its task in a different way, each has a set of shared objectives:

- Promoting local community interests in the NHS
- Promoting improved quality in health services
- Providing a link between the NHS and the public
- Promoting individual rights.

The CHCs' Patients' Charter

In 1986 the Association of Community Health Councils produced its 'Patients' Charter' of basic rights for people in healthcare[3]. It was based on the experience of member CHCs and was presented as a set of guidelines for good practice in NHS care.

The guidelines state that all persons have a right to:

- Health services appropriate to their need, regardless of financial needs or where they live and without delay
- Be treated with reasonable skill, care and consideration (Both these were already an established legal right)
- Written information about health services, including hospitals, community and general practioner services
- Register with a general practioner with ease and be able to change without adverse consequences
- Be informed about all aspects of their condition and proposed care (including alternatives available) unless they express a wish to the contrary
- Accept or refuse treatment (including diagnostic procedures), without affecting the standard of alternative care given
- A second opinion
- The support of a relative or a friend at any time
- Advocacy and interpreting services (see below)

41

- Choose whether to participate or not in research trials and be free to withdraw at any time without affecting the standard of alternative care given

- Be discharged from hospital only after adequate arrangements have been made for their continuing care

- Privacy for all consultations, confidentiality of all records relating to their care, and access to their own healthcare records

- Be treated at all times with respect for their dignity, personal needs and religious and philosophical beliefs

- Make a complaint and have it investigated thoroughly, speedily and be informed of the result

- An independent investigation into all serious medical or other mishaps while in NHS care, whether or not a complaint is made, and, where appropriate, adequate redress.

ACTIVITY 4
discussion
Compare the Association of Community Health Councils' Patients' Charter with the government's *Patient's Charter* (see *P1(ii): Health and power* for information about the government's *Patient's Charter*). Note any similarities and differences that you find. How easy do you think it would be to implement both sets of guidelines in your workplace? You may wish to discuss this with some of your colleagues.

Advocacy

Advocacy is acting on behalf of, and in the best interests of, an individual or group who are unable to act for themselves. Their inability to do so may be because they do not realise that they can do so, because they lack information or are in a position of fear, or because they lack the required skills.

EXAMPLE

An interesting example of advocacy was implemented by City and Hackney CHC, in inner London, which was concerned about the delivery of healthcare to non-English speaking women. Many had difficulty in communicating their problems and finding their way through the system. The CHC employed a health worker as 'patients' advocate'. The aims of the project were to:

- Improve access to health services

- Help women to understand choices open to them so that they could make informed decisions

- Advise the health authority on policy and practice with regard to the needs of non-English speaking women

- Help and encourage NHS staff to provide a service to non-English speaking women.

A subsequent study in 1984 showed improvements in take-up in antenatal care, in nutrional status of the mothers and in their babies' birth-weights, which can be attributed to the project. No trends were found in the control group of English-speaking women, except an increase in non-attendance at antenatal clinics[4].

ACTIVITY 5
discussion
Now read the report you obtained for Activity 3 and note down, in relation to the Association of CHCs' Patients' Charter, any points in the report you personally feel are important. This will depend on your interests. If you are working in a group you could compare notes and devise a list of important points reflecting a range of interests.

Self-help Groups

In recent years, community health councils have been active in helping people to make and resolve complaints against a trust. A number of self-help groups have been formed.

A self-help group is a group of people who share a similar experience or problem. They now exist in many walks of life, including women's and ethnic groups, and have come into being to help, support and provide information for their members and for other interested or relevant people. Self-help groups may also provide members with emotional support, material assistance, friendship and technical expertise. In addition, they may offer an emotional refuge from discrimination and stigma[5], and some, such as MENCAP, also act as political pressure groups to campaign for support for their members.

It can be argued that self-help is a response to the decline of existing social institutions such as the churches and extended family. It is also a useful means of bringing attention to particular problems of healthcare, by bringing together many small voices into a more powerful consumer group.

Nurses and Self-help

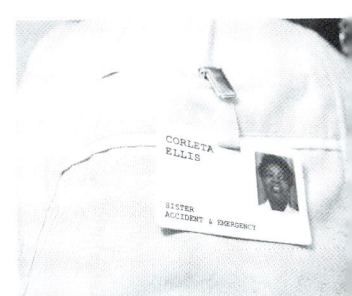

Oakley[6] argues that nurses should heed the consumer healthcare movement and amend their practice by taking consumer views into account. Certainly, the Labour Government is keen to ensure that the consumer has more of a voice in the way healthcare is provided. It is not unusual, for example, for a community health council representative to be a non-voting member of an NHS trust board.

National self-help groups are listed in national directories. A useful one is *The Voluntary Agencies Directory*[7]. Even a casual glance through such a directory reveals an amazing variety of special health interests. A list of local groups can be found in public libraries or obtained from your local Council for Voluntary Service. If you send for any information from a voluntary organisation remember to enclose a stamped self-addressed envelope, as postage is a major expense for them.

ACTIVITY 6
action
• Write down a list of all the national and local self-help groups which are relevant to your nursing practice.
• Send off for the news/information sheet of those groups which you think would be most useful to you.

Should nurses play an active part in self-help groups rather than playing a more passive learning role? Jertson[8] queries active professional involvement in self-help groups because of fear that this might detract from the ability of a self-help group to do just that. Too deep an involvement may also mean that the professional rapidly takes the role of the 'expert' and ceases to learn from the group. Much valuable insight that could have been taken into nursing practice would thus be lost. Professionals should seek to learn from self-help groups and not to lead or teach them.

The Royal College of Nursing Commission on the National Health Service and Health Care has no doubt that consumers' voices are not heard, describing them as 'probably the weakest and least powerful actors on the health service stage'[9].

ACTIVITY 7
action
If you feel that attending a meeting of a relevant self-help group would add to your understanding, contact the group leader, explain why you would like to go along, and ask how the group would feel about your being there. If you are invited to a meeting be careful that your professional role does not take over the meeting!

The Commission believes that all parts of the health service must alter their procedures and attitudes to facilitate the development of consumer opportunities and choices. However, although change overall may come gradually, there is nothing to stop each of us taking immediate personal action to ensure that we listen to consumers' voices. This means that, in addition to listening when they manage to make themselves heard, we go out of our way to seek their opinions. This is why we suggest contacting self-help groups.

Notes

The relationship between healthcare professional and patient is changing. It is now recognised that clients want greater control over their care, treatment and social support. In response to the government's 1997 consultation paper, *Towards the 21st Century: The way forward for the NHS*[10], the NHS Confederation stressed that:

'Citizens' demands for a bigger say in the direction of health policy are leading to greater openness and explicitness by public bodies given stewardship of taxpayers' money. This will be exacerbated by the increasing need for difficult decisions to be made concerning priorities for health and healthcare, where consumer demand and medical technological advance are outstripping the system's ability to deliver to meet population expectations'.

ACTIVITY 8
discussion
Write down the key points from your visit(s) to the self-help group(s). Discuss them with your work colleagues. Make a note of the comments made by the group and any conclusions you reach.

FEEDBACK

If you have been able to reach any conclusion on action to be taken to take consumer opinions into account, such as regularly receiving a particular self-help group's news sheets, you will have gone some way as a group to taking the consumer view in your nursing practice. If your group was not convinced, or if you work alone, there is still a very important point to consider.

The nursing profession is not an official body like the United Kingdom Central Council for Nursing, Midwifery and Health Visiting, the national boards or the Royal College of Nursing. It is thousands of people like us, and it is up to each one of us to take action to ensure that consumer opinions of health and illness, and of the care appropriate for each individual, are heard.

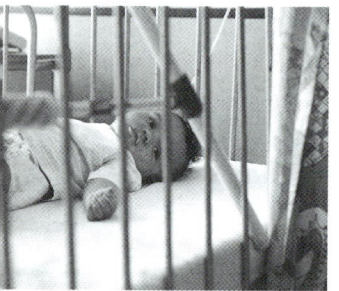

FOCUS

Write a brief report (about one page) outlining the actions you plan to take consumer opinion into account in your professional practice, and give reasons why you have decided to take this action.

REFERENCES

1. Illich, I. *Disabling Professions.* London: Marion Boyars, 1977.
2. Murcott, A. Health as ideology. In: Atkinson, P., Dingwall, R., Murcott, A. *Prospects for the National Health.* London: Croom Helm, 1979.
3. Association of Community Health Councils for England and Wales. *Patients' Charter.* London: ACHC 1986.
4. Hogg, C. *Good Practices in CHCs.* London: Association of Community Health Councils for England and Wales, 1988.
5. Henry, S., Robinson, D. The self-help way to health. In: Atkinson, P., Dingwall, R., Murcott, A. *Prospects for the National Health.* London: Croom Helm, 1979.
6. Oakley, A. What price professionalism? The importance of being a nurse. *Nursing Times* 1984; **80**: 50,24-27.
7. *The Voluntary Agencies Directory.* London: NCVO Publishers, 1998.
8. Jertson, J. Self-help groups. *Social Work* 1975; **20**: 144–145.
9. The Commission on the National Health Service and Health Care in the United Kingdom (Chairman: J. Neuberger). *The Health Challenge: A report of a Commission on the National Health Services and Health Care in the United Kingdom established by the Royal College of Nursing.* London: RCN, 1988.
10. NHS Confederation. *Towards the 21st Century. The way forward for the NHS.* (Consultation Paper.) Birmingham: NHS Confederation. (Tel: 0121 471 4444.)

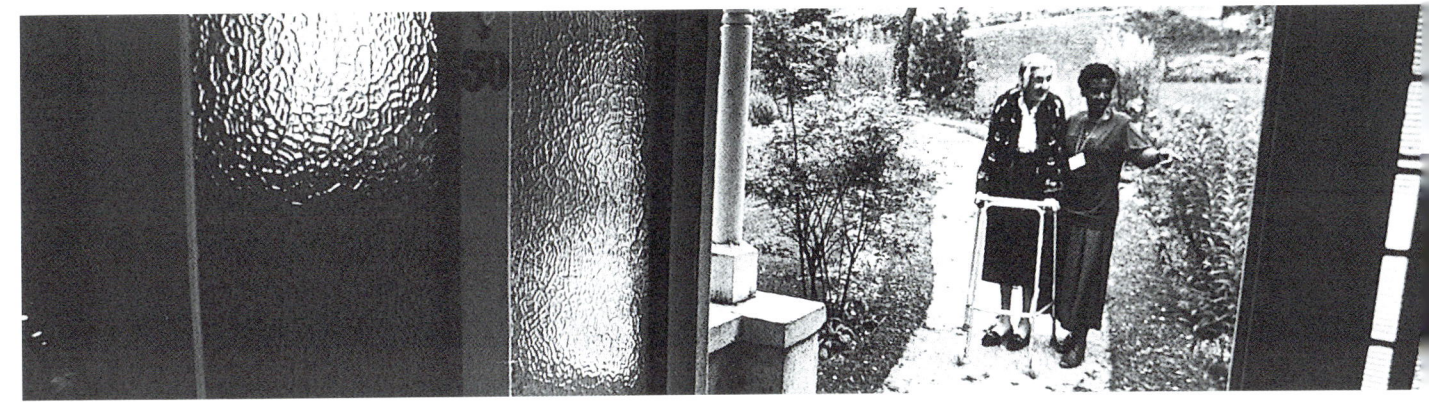

A personal approach

What do you hear when clients give you details about themselves? What assumptions do you make about what they are telling you?

This Part considers:

- Attitudes associated with the community you grew up in and how your views may change over time

- Milestones in your life

- The use of lifelines.

Through the Activities, you may discover how your own view of the world colours the way you view others. *P2(ii): Different lives, different perspectives* looks at the way other people's view of the world is different from our own and prepares the ground for a later Section, *P5: Client Assessment*, which considers practical ways in which increased understanding of ourselves and others can help improve standards of care.

WORK PLANNER

The Focus Activity asks you to interview someone over the age of 70 about his/her life history. Try to carry out the interview and follow-up before you start work on *P2(ii): Different lives, different perspectives*, as it will provide useful preparation for what is to come. If this is not possible, arrange for the interview to take place as soon as possible, and do all the preparation work now.

Read through the Focus first, and make sure that you are clear about what you are asked to do. If possible, choose someone who is related to you, or whom you know quite well, and avoid approaching anyone who is undergoing any form of life crisis (such as illness or bereavement). Explain about the course, and why you want to carry out the interview and then ASK THE PERSON'S PERMISSION TO DO SO. You will find more information about conducting interviews in your student pack.

Activity 8 asks you to construct your lifeline, based on the major world events which have occurred in your lifetime. The best concise reference source for events of the 20th century is *Pears Cyclopaedia*, published annually by Penguin books. An up-to-date edition should be available in any library reference section.

THE BIOGRAPHICAL APPROACH

Whatever kind of nursing setting you work in, you will, in the course of your work, collect large amounts of information about the individuals in your care.

Nursing documentation usually includes such headings as name, age, address, next of kin, present or former occupation, religion, and past medical history. This kind of information is

45

collected and recorded to meet immediate practical needs — for example: who should be contacted in the event of an emergency; is the person subjected to any hazardous conditions at work; are there any special needs arising from the person's religious affiliation?

But such information can also have another important function in determining the quality of nursing care.

> **ACTIVITY 1**
> **diary**
> Have you ever thought about what other purpose a client's personal history could serve in helping you provide better nursing care? Stop reading and consider this for a few minutes, then jot down your ideas in your diary.

In nursing, we aim to provide care which meets the needs of every individual. Yet such individualised care is possible only if we can see beyond labels which emphasise what people have in common — a heart condition, or a mental illness, for example — and recognise their essential individuality.

A person's *biography* — his or her life history — is as distinctive as that person's fingerprints. As explained in *P1(i): A personal view of health and illness*, people's experience of life determines the way they perceive their health — how good it is, when it is under threat, and when to seek advice. It will also affect the way they view healthcare and the people who provide it. Understanding the origins of different people's attitudes to health and illness is an important element in our approach to a client, and in the next two Parts we will explore how we can increase this understanding.

We're going to start off, as we will many times in this course, by looking at *you*.

WHERE ARE YOU COMING FROM?

Understanding your past is a major step in understanding your attitudes and responses to other people.

'Where you are coming from' is not just where you started, but all the places you have been on the way. Let's start by thinking about your beginnings, about what influenced you in your childhood.

> **ACTIVITY 2**
> **diary**
> Think about where you grew up and make some notes about the sort of community you grew up in. By community we mean the people you grew up with, played with, went to school with, and their families. Can you describe the attitudes of this community towards:
> • Children • Old people • Work • Sex • Death
> • Unmarried mothers • Working mothers
> • Divorce • Marriage • People from other cultures
> • Religion • Illness • Health
> • Handicap
> Write a sentence or two in your diary about each. Remember to write in the part of your diary which is confidential.

In thinking about this Activity, you may have uncovered some things you had almost forgotten — attitudes, biases and traditions which are still part of you and which affect the way you think and feel about others.

ACTIVITY 3
diary
Look again at your responses to the list in Activity 2. Which attitudes of the community you grew up in are still part of your life now?
What other events or experiences in your life have had a significant influence on your attitudes? You may be able to identify particular things which happened to you personally, or a national or international event which added a new dimension to your outlook on life. Examples may be becoming a parent for the first time, a personal bereavement or the death of a world figure, changes in legislation, or taxation, or a particular story which hit the headlines and which has changed your perspective on life.

FEEDBACK

Activities 2 and 3 may have helped you to identify where some of your attitudes and views have come from. New experiences and events shape our attitudes and views throughout our lives.

ACTIVITY 4
diary
Now return to the list in Activity 2 and make a few notes about your own attitude to each of those topics. Your experience of life, along with the changes that have taken place in society since you were a child, may well mean that you have very different views now.

By doing these Activities, we hope that you will have begun to see how your own background colours the way in which you view the lives of others. You can begin to recognise how other people, with different childhood and life experiences, will be coming from a different direction.

A SHARED PAST

Now let us look at some of the things you have met on your way through life.

ACTIVITY 5
discussion
Think about the 10 most important events in your life — the things which are most important to you personally. Jot them down in your diary. When you get the chance, ask two or three other people, friends or colleagues, to do the same thing. Compare notes with other members of your study group.

FEEDBACK

We would guess that, although the nature of events might differ widely, most people would choose the same sorts of events as *milestones* in their life — going to school, leaving school, graduating or completing training, getting married, giving birth to children, and so on.

These events form the framework of our shared background. We can share on an individual basis; for example, if we know people who are parents, and they have this in common with us, our attitude towards them may be different from what it would be towards those who are not parents. Similarly, if we know someone is a nurse, we can share things that we could not share with others.

These milestones also shape the way we behave in groups — whether they be small social groups, or larger groups, such as the community which you considered in Activity 2. Each one of us belongs to a number of such groups — for example, our nationality, our profession, or our friends; all set the boundaries of different groups that we belong to at one time.

Every group has its own particular shared knowledge, which determines the assumptions we make about people within the group and outside it. Again, being part of a group, with its shared knowledge, colours the way we look at people who are outside the group.

Notes

**ACTIVITY 6
diary**
Try to describe your own social group — the people with whom you interact as a part of your everyday life. How does this social group differ from the community that you considered in Activity 2? Jot down the attitude of your social group towards the things we listed in Activity 2.

In this Activity we have started to think about the mutual knowledge of our own particular social group, and have added another dimension to the way we view other people.

Beyond the shared knowledge of our own particular group, there are also things that we share with many more people.

**ACTIVITY 7
discussion**
Now make a list of what you think are the 10 most important events which have happened in the world during your lifetime. How many of these have affected you directly, and how? For those which have not affected you directly, say why you think they are important.
Compare your list with those of others in your student group. It might highlight some interesting differences. Can you identify the reasons for these differences?

A BIOGRAPHICAL MODEL

From the information you have gained from Activities 2–7, it is possible to construct a simple model which illustrates the way in which your personal history, or biography, is built up (see Figure 1).

Fig. 1. A biographical model

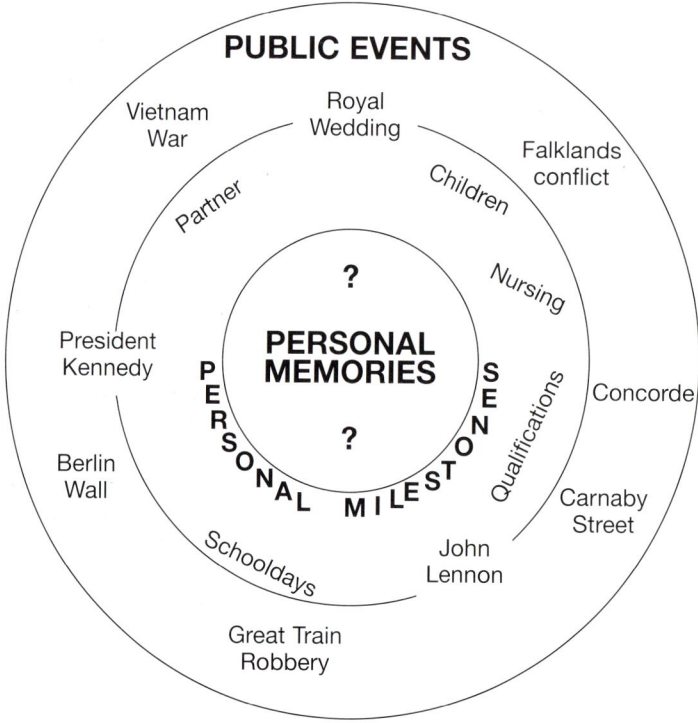

A *model* is a way of organising our knowledge about some aspect of reality, to give us a means of making comparisons and of testing ideas we might have about the way things are. In a later Section in the programme *(P11): Models for Care*, we will be looking at some of the models which are used as the basis for the organisation of nursing care.

The model illustrated in Fig. 1 gives you a snapshot of your own life history or biography. This is a way of organising the information you have assembled in your work so far this week.

At the centre of the model are the personal experiences and memories which have shaped you as an individual. They are the most important part of your biography, the things you thought about in Activities 2 and 3.

The second ring of the model shows *personal milestones*, experiences which mark our belonging to a group. These form part of our shared past.

On the outside of the model are *public events* — events in the outside world which register in some way in our personal history. Although they usually have no direct effect on us, they are links with the past which we all share.

We want to use this model as a starting point from which to explore some of the factors which may cause others, and in particular our clients, to have a very different view of the world, and of us and the care we provide. *P2(ii) Different lives, different perspectives* considers ways in which we can understand these views in order to be able to provide appropriate care for all our clients, and Activity 8 is intended to prepare the ground for that work.

ACTIVITY 8
diary
Using a blank page in your diary, draw your lifeline. Draw a vertical line down the page, creating two columns. At the top of the left-hand column mark WORLD EVENTS. Divide the column into decades starting with the year of your birth at the top of the column, and ending with 1990 at the bottom of the column. List the major world events which have taken place in each decade. Mark the right-hand column PERSONAL MEMORIES. In this column make a note of your memories of those events. A sample lifeline for someone who was born in 1900 is shown on the next page.

Drawing a lifeline like this helps to highlight and compare our experiences of public events. For example, for one person a Royal Wedding may be a vivid adult memory; for another it may be just a hazy recollection of a day's holiday from school.

Someone from a different cultural background to your own may also have a completely different perspective on what were important world events during a particular decade.

ACTIVITY 9
discussion
Compare your lifeline with those of the other students in your group. Discuss the reasons for any differences. Can you identify the factors which caused people to have different lifelines? You might also find it interesting to get members of different generations in your family to do lifelines and compare notes.

A Lifeline to the Past

	World events	Personal memories
1900	Birth of Labour Party Queen Victoria died King Edward VII crowned	My mother took me to watch the coronation procession — I remember a lot of noise, flags, and the horses.
1910	First World War Suffragette movement	Ran away at 16 to join up — they brought me back, but I joined up two years later. My father was killed in France.
1920	King George's jubilee Flappers/Charleston Wall Street crash Depression/unemployment	After demob things weren't very good. I had no job. We didn't have much — no one round our way did — though I'm sure some people managed to make money. We couldn't afford to get married.
1930	Abdication of Edward VIII Second World War broke out	We got married two years after I got a job — had two kids. When the King decided to go, I thought he was mad.
1940	War years Welfare State Rationing Marriage of Princess Elizabeth	Wounded in the Western Desert — spent most of the time in field hospitals — awful they were — couldn't even get fags most of the time. I was sent home. D-day was wonderful. My older son got diphtheria in 1949, but thanks to the new Welfare State he was OK.
1950	End of rationing Suez crisis Coronation Korean War	We had a street party to celebrate the coronation. I was sick at the time — chronic bronchitis, they said. I remember the Suez Crisis — thought my boy might get called up. My brother emigrated to Australia.
1960	Kennedy assassination Cuba crisis Berlin Wall erected Beatlemania/flower power Man on the moon	I was in hospital when we heard the news about Kennedy — Sister let us keep the radios on to hear about it. My chest got worse, so I never went back to work. Went to son's house to watch the moon landing with my grandchildren.
1970	Miners' strike/three-day week War in Vietnam Watergate Britain joins EEC Irish troubles escalate	Power cuts had us sitting in the dark with no TV — my wife was ill, and it didn't make life any easier. Oil prices went up, and so did our heating bills. President Nixon resigned — always though he was a bit tricky myself. The IRA started bombing in London — didn't worry me though — don't go up to town any more.
1980	Margaret Thatcher Falklands Chernobyl Reagan/Gorbachev End of Berlin Wall	Our boys won in the Falklands — though my grandson says the whole thing was a waste of money. I've been waiting a year to go into hospital — it's getting harder and harder to walk — but they just keep saying, 'It's the cuts'.

The Focus Activity asks you to carry out a biographical interview with someone who is over the age of 70, to look at that person's lifeline and begin to consider how one factor — age — might affect a person's view of the past, and his or her attitudes and expectations of health and health care. These ideas are followed up in *P2(ii): Different lives, different perspectives.*

FOCUS

The aim of this interview is to gather biographical information about someone much older than you. Once you have this information you can draw the person's lifeline, using the same model you created in Activity 8.

Preparation

Before you interview the person you have selected, make a rough plan of what you want to ask:

(a) The person's perceptions of the public events

(b) The person's personal milestones.

The interview

You won't want to make your interview too formal, but try to remember all the things you planned to ask. We suggest that during the interview you listen carefully and respond, and jot down the person's memories of their lifetime.

Try to explore beyond the biographical details by asking questions about personal milestones in the context of the public events you have outlined (for example: 'What can you remember of public events in the first 10 years of your life? The first 20?' 'How did the depression affect your childhood?' 'What was it like getting married during the War?'). Be wary about trying to pry too far — you may be getting close to the core of your subject's memories, those which he or she might not wish to share.

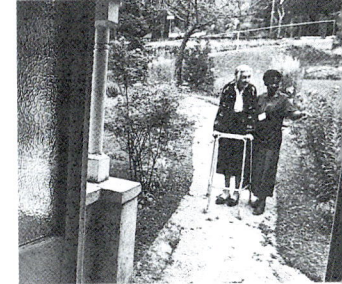

Follow-up

As soon as possible after the interview, make some concise notes in your diary about what was said. In particular, note any differences in attitude between yourself and the person you interviewed towards things you have both experienced (such as education, illness or marriage). Can you explain these differences?

Did the simple model we described on page 48 seem to apply to your respondent's recall of biographical detail?

Did the interview reveal anything about the attitudes of an older person towards your shared past which surprised you?

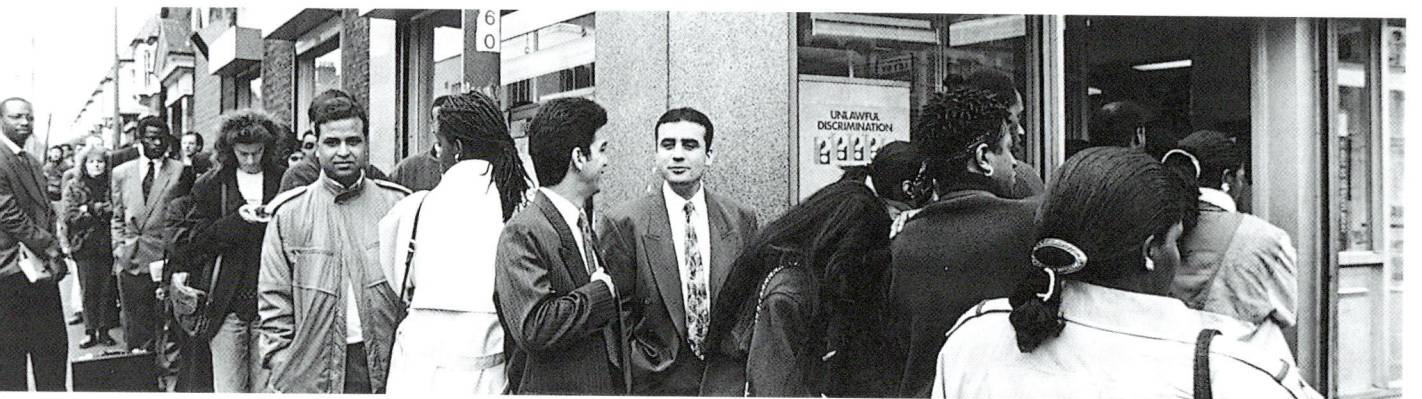

Different lives, different perspectives

P2(i): A personal approach looked at your own biography — the events which have shaped your own personal history and how this colours the way you view other people. This Part explores the ways in which people from different backgrounds may have different views and expectations of healthcare.

Key points covered in this Part are:

- How age influences the perspective of people on the subject of healthcare

- Our attitudes towards people from different cultural backgrounds and what their health-care needs are

- The perspective of people facing life in the community after a long period in an institution.

WORK PLANNER

In Activity 2 you will look at health care in your area before the establishment of the NHS. You will need to visit a library to find this information.

WHO FITS THE PICTURE?

Many nurses are able to construct an 'identikit' picture of their typical patient or client.

EXAMPLE

For a nurse working in a trauma ward, most patients might be local men, under the age of 30, who have been involved in road traffic accidents, or accidents involving hazardous sports. Similarly, in a unit for the elderly mentally ill, most clients will be over the age of 70, and will be suffering from depression or one of the forms of dementia.

ACTIVITY 1
diary

Think for a few moments about your patients or clients. Then take your diary and list down the left of the page the main features of personal history which might be shared by a 'typical' individual under your care. Then think about those clients who do not share the background you have outlined and, on the right of the page, make a list of the factors which make them 'atypical' (not typical) or 'different'. How do you deal with these 'atypical' factors when providing healthcare? Feel free to make an honest assessment. Do you try to ignore the differences, to treat all your patients and clients the same? If not, how do you try to cater for the differences?

FEEDBACK

Your list of biographical elements which make some of your clients different might include social background, ethnic or cultural background, age, an unusual disease or a nursing problem.

Our society operates on the basis of broad assumptions about large groups of people — for example, that all nurses are women, or that all nurses are general nurses. While these statements may be true of the majority, they can easily obscure the identity of minority groups.

As well as emphasising what people have in common — childhood memories, their first job — personal histories have an important role to play in providing clues to individual differences. Here, we will look at some of the biographical factors which may make clients different from one another, and explore our own attitudes to these factors.

THE AGE FACTOR

The Focus in *P2(i): A personal approach* encouraged an insight into how old people may have a view of the past, and the important moments in their lives, which differ from your own.

P1(i): A personal view of health and illness looked at the case of Albert, and how attitudes to health were very much shaped by his age. His background, and the attitudes to health and illness (and to 'cripples' in particular) of the culture in which he grew up, shaped his attitude to his own needs for healthcare.

But a person's age can determine other things as well. Let's explore how the length of a person's lifeline can influence perceptions of health.

For those of us born after 1948, and the creation of the Welfare State and the National Health Service, it is easy to forget that older people may have very different memories of healthcare, and that these may affect their attitudes to the current health service.

This is one woman's account of an operation carried out in 1912[1]:

> 'I was 12 years of age ... the operation was done on the kitchen table. The nurse came and the doctor and I've so much of my rib taken, it's cut down here and down my back and it was done on the kitchen table. The nurse came and attended to the wound for seven weeks. They gave me an anaesthetic. All had to take place during the housework and the older ones coming in for their meals ... The doctor said: "Mrs R, this is ideal for the job; you couldn't have had a better table". There was no talk of going into hospital, and it was just done at home.'

Do you remember any preparations beforehand?

> 'There was no walls scrubbed, but everything had to be clean and I remember mother saying that the nurse said: "Well, you've got everything just right." They had a bucket at the end to hold the blood.'

There are still many people who can remember the era of the Poor Law, with the stigma that became attached to entering the workhouse as a pauper. The provisions of the Poor Law, which dated back to Elizabethan times, were finally abolished in 1929, when local government took over responsibility for the poor from 'guardians' elected by the parish and community.

53

For some older people, a nursing interview may bring back unhappy memories of a former interview with healthcare officials. Applicants for help under the Poor Law first had to convince the relieving officer that their need was genuine, and this hated means test is remembered to this day[2]:

'If a man couldn't get a job he'd go round to the RO, it used to be Mary Anne's buildings, to see the Relieving Officer. His name was Mr Abbot and he was a very hard man. If he thought that a man didn't want to work, he'd say, "Oh well, you can't find work, so you and your wife will have to go in the workhouse." The father went one place, the mother and the children somewhere else.'

ACTIVITY 2
knowledge base
Find out about how health care was provided in your area before the establishment of the NHS in 1948. Where were the main hospitals, mental institutions, and so on? The librarian at your college of nursing or public library will probably be able to help you find this information. Ask one or two older members of the community whether they can remember if any institutions had a particular stigma attached to them. How do you think that a knowledge of the history of a particular hospital, perhaps one which was formerly a workhouse, might affect an older person's attitude to being cared for in it?

It's not just older people whose perceptions of health and illness are affected by their age. Other age groups, too, are likely to have certain assumptions and attitudes. Let's look at two examples of the way in which people's age affects their attitude to illness and health care.

EXAMPLES

People's age — not just whether they are old — will be a factor in relation to the way an illness affects their working lives. For some patients, a condition requiring nursing care is simply a brief interlude in a busy and fulfilling career. For others, their illness may create the prospect of having to find a less demanding job, or leaving employment altogether. Older clients may be coming to terms with retirement, and the loss of job satisfaction, income or status that this often involves.

Age may also influence the way clients see you, and hence the sort of relationship you have with them. Consider the practice of calling clients by their first name. This may help to foster a good relationship with someone who is of a similar age to you, but how do you think an older person might feel about it?

Many older people use more formal language ('Mr' or 'Mrs') with people of their own age whom they have known for years. They have no choice but to call you 'Nurse', and they may feel that they are being patronised, or 'talked down to' if you use first names and they cannot. This might contribute to a feeling of helplessness, and of their having no control over their situation.

ACTIVITY 3
diary
Think about the examples above. Do any of the statements made there apply to your relationship with any of your clients? Had you thought of this before? If not, note in your diary how it might affect the care you provide.

In this Section we have been working towards a better understanding of how people's age can affect their attitude to health and illness. If you can introduce this understanding into healthcare, you will give your clients a greater feeling of control over their own health and healthcare.

This notion of control is especially important when considering different cultural groups.

IN A STRANGE LAND

Britain is a multicultural society. Many people have come to this country since the 1950s from the New Commonwealth, but there are also large groups of migrants who came, for example, from Eastern Europe before and during the Second World War to escape persecution by the Nazis[3].

Whatever the motive — whether political or economic — most migrants came to Britain with high hopes for the future.

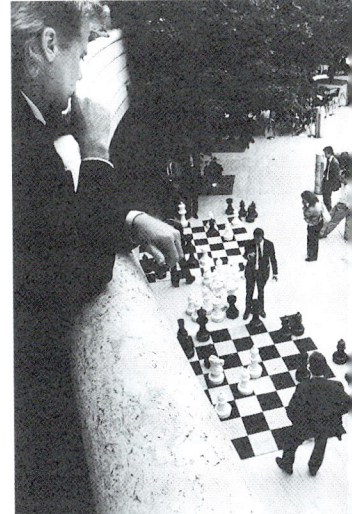

However, although what they found was in many ways an improvement on what they had left (safety from persecution, or more job opportunities), for many, Britain has been a disappointing place. Despite the fact that many migrant families have been here for over 30 years, they still experience a general feeling of exclusion.

Ethnic minorities are sometimes seen as a 'problem' politically and socially[3]. Although racial discrimination is illegal in Britain, many individuals and groups in British society do discriminate against those from other cultures. This racism permeates to healthcare, how it is provided, and how it is 'perceived' by minority groups.

Racism does not need to be malevolent for it to be effective. Much racism is by omission (what we *don't* do) rather than commission (what we *do* do) — people simply don't think about the differing needs of the various ethnic communities.

ACTIVITY 4
diary
What is your own attitude to people from different cultural groups to your own? Do you discriminate against such people by omission (what you don't do to take their views and needs into account)? Share your thoughts with your diary.

Many people find it quite difficult to be completely honest, even with themselves, about their views on people from other racial groups. However, most of us, if we were completely truthful, would find elements of racism in ourselves, whatever cultural group we belong to.

What we have to do as nurses is to see beyond the prejudice to some of the problems it presents for us in practice. We want our clients to feel comfortable with the care we provide, to feel they have some control over their own health and the treatment they receive. We are now going to consider what additional biographical details will help to give us the insight we need to help ethnic minority groups get more out of the healthcare system.

Each different group will have different cultural 'filters' through which they view the healthcare services which this country provides — different attitudes, for example, to religion, the family, the role of women, care for the elderly and for those with learning disabilities. How can we explore these 'filters' further to increase our understanding of our clients' needs?

P2(i): A personal approach used the concept of a lifeline to show how a person's age can colour his or her view of life. Now consider what the lifeline of someone born in another part of the world might look like. In the 1940s, many Ukrainian and Yugoslav immigrants who came from displaced persons camps in liberated Germany included workers who had been forcibly recruited by the Nazi regime to work in Germany's industry and agriculture under harsh conditions[4]. The following illustration uses a group of Ukrainian migrants in Bradford, researched by Robert Perks. It shows how, once a community becomes established in Britain, there is a complex period of acclimatisation as succeeding generations try to establish a balance between their original backgrounds and their British identities.

'I born for Ukraine country, I like my country, I want to go back my country. If my country free.'

1st generation Ukrainian, aged 74

Q. 'You say you have an English passport and you have got English nationality. Do you still see yourself, though, as Ukrainian?'

A. 'I do, it sounds odd, but I really do: I would never say anything against the British and I mean they have given me everything, and they have given me an education and so on and so forth, but in my heart I just feel Ukrainian; you know it is really odd.'

2nd generation Ukrainian, aged 34

Q. 'Do you think you will ever go to the Ukraine?'

A. 'Yes, I'd like to go when I'm older.'

Q. 'Yes — why would you like to go?'

A. 'Well, I have never seen it, and I'm kind of part of it, so I'd like to go and see it, and see my relations there.'

3rd generation Ukrainian, aged 10

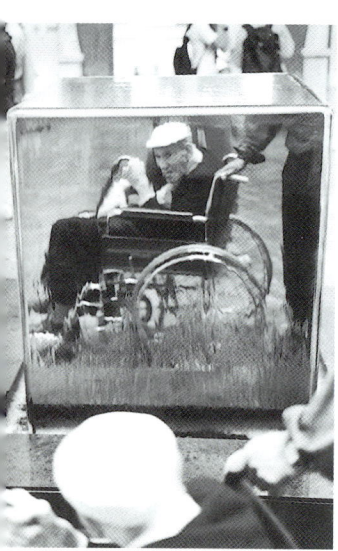

ACTIVITY 5
diary
In your diary, list the major factors which might influence the attitude towards healthcare of each of the people quoted above. Choose an example of a factor which influences health, such as diet, and jot down how the attitudes of each generation might differ.

Each of these three generations has a different cultural filter, which gives them different views of many aspects of life, including healthcare.

The elderly Ukrainian in our example still sees himself as being of a different nationality to the country in which he lives. His attitudes to healthcare will probably be drawn from the traditions of his own cultural group, as well as from his experience of living in a foreign land for 50 years. His attitude to diet might be determined by Ukrainian traditions of cooking, and strongly influenced by periods of hardship and shortage.

The second-generation migrant will have a mixture of influences — the traditional culture will have been diluted somewhat, and the British culture, with its belief in the welfare state, will not be alien to him. People of this generation may be in a position to draw strengths from both of the cultures they represent. His parents' views and practices on diet will exert a strong influence, but he has lived through a period of great change in what is available to the British diet, so his views may have changed considerably during his life.

For the third-generation migrant, probably almost totally integrated into British society, the traditions and values of Ukrainian society may seem distant. If and when he ever makes his visit, he will find that they, too, have changed. His views on diet will be shaped more by his peer group at school, and the pressures created by advertising than by the traditions of his grandfathers.

You will begin to see how biographical details become even more important when different cultural backgrounds are involved. We will be returning to this theme many times throughout the course, but we would like you to spend some time in this Part reflecting on the different cultural groups you meet during your nursing practice.

ACTIVITY 6
diary
Write down the different cultural
groups with which you come into
contact during your nursing practice.
Make a note of the ways in which the healthcare
system in which you work discriminates against
people from other cultures. For example, in an area
with a large Islamic population, should the concerns
of Moslem women for privacy and modesty be met
by the provision of more women doctors?
Should translation services be available for
non-English speakers? During certain times
or 24 hours a day?
What factors need to be taken into
account when deciding how far the
needs of any one group can
be catered for?

ACTIVITY 7
discussion
Discuss your thoughts from
Activity 6 with colleagues,
managers, and other healthcare professionals with whom
you come into contact. What
is the general view?
You may want to make
some notes in
your diary.

HIDDEN LIVES

The following are extracts from an article about the personal histories of residents in one, not necessarily typical, mental handicap hospital who now face the prospect of life in the community[5]:

Some people's memories vividly recapture the fear, bewilderment and helplessness most people, at whatever level of comprehension, must have felt at being 'put away' in such a large, depersonalising place:

'My grandfather didn't say where I was going. That's what got me, he didn't say where. Frightened I were. I felt awful! I wanted to go back out. I felt upset! I couldn't stick it in here!'

However, some found it harder to recall and articulate their feelings — not just in relation to admission, but more generally. In commenting on painful experiences and various deprivations such as the lack of personal possessions, birthday celebrations, friendships or visits from relatives, people would sometimes say: 'I didn't bother.' Inherent difficulties interpreting and describing feelings may well have been compounded by the fact that institutions did not encourage or expect inmates to need to do so. Pretending not to feel or not to mind must, for some, have become an automatic and effective method of coping with the pain of neglect ...

The system exercised complete control and tyranny over the inmates through reward and punishment. Work pay/pocket money, visits to and from home, holidays and recreational activities were considered privileges that had to be earned by 'good conduct and work', as one man illustrates:

'Patients had to be careful how they behaved in their work and the villa or wherever they were 'cos there was strict staff in those days, and any offence they used to be up before one of the senior doctors. In the case of first offences, they were warned of the serious nature of the offence and what would happen if that or anything like it was repeated. Then they were placed before the doctor and they lost all their privileges for a certain length of time ... Privileges were ... going to films and concerts and in hospital grounds, recreation hall and money included.'

More severe punishments, both official and unofficial such as cold baths, scrubbing, carrying bags of sand and beatings existed for those who more openly rebelled against the system ...

cont ...

Notes

... cont

'If you got caught doing summat to a girl they used to lock you up in a side-room ... without no clothes on.'

One woman who has lived in the hospital since she was six remembered the darker side of institutional life:

'You know, if we did something wrong we had to be in us nighties all day and be punished. Couldn't go out anywhere, couldn't have your visitors to see you. If you were bursting to go somewhere and you wet yourself, you know like with me, you got punished. Say you were in a wheelchair and you couldn't talk to tell them, you still got punished!

'I didn't like it [food] and we used to grumble and groan, but if we didn't eat it for your tea, they'd save it for your supper. You had to eat it and eat it and eat it 'til it were gone! We daren't leave anything, them days.'

Despite this woman's apparent satisfaction with life and improvements in the system, she could admit that she felt she had lived in the institution too long once she become more secure and confident:

'Now I've started going home, I'm a lot happier. I never used to go home or anything. It was alright then (in the old days). I think it was nice and alright. I hadn't been here long enough then, but now I'm thinking I've been at The Park too long now. I wish I would leave in one way. I don't mean to be nasty. I'd like to go and see somewhere, you know, nice places. Would they let us have a change? I'm just getting a bit fed up of being here. You know I've been here a long time. Are they supposed to be building some houses? I hope I'm not going to stay here much longer!'

ACTIVITY 8
diary
What sort of lifeline do you think people who have lived in institutions for a long time might have? Write brief notes in your diary about what the extracts from the article quoted above reveal about the needs of residents of mental hospitals as they face the prospect of life in the community.

The examples we have looked at here illustrate how the detail of people's lives (including our own) affects their perceptions of other people. Understanding more about how others see us as well as how we see other people will help us provide the best care for our clients.

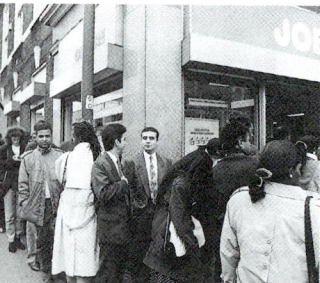

FOCUS

Look back at the answers you gave to Activity 1. Consider your view of your clients' differences. How could you improve the way you provide healthcare for your diverse range of clients in the future?

REFERENCES

1. Roberts, E. A. M. *Working Class Barrow and Lancaster 1890–1930.* Occasional Paper No. 2. Lancaster: Centre for North-West Regional Studies, University of Lancaster, 1976.
2. Birkett, J. In: Schweitzer, P. (eds.) *Can We Afford the Doctor?* Blackheath: Age Exchange, 1985.
3. Coxall, B., Robins, L. *Contemporary British Politics.* London: Macmillan, 1989; 438.
4. Perks, R. B. A feeling of not belonging: Interviewing European immigrants in Bradford. *Oral History* 1984; **12**: 2, 64–67.
5. Fido R., Potts, M. 'It's not true what was written down': Experiences of life in a mental handicap institution. *Oral History* 1989; **17**: 2, 31–34.

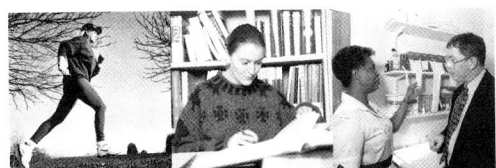

Term 2

In Term 1 our focus was on the attitudes and views of individuals towards healthcare and nursing. In Term 2 we broaden the focus to explore the wider framework of healthcare and the role of the nursing profession, and you as an individual member of it.

The first Section (P3) explores the environment in which healthcare is provided, and discusses issues of public and individual responsibility in maintaining the nation's health.

The second Section (R2) returns to the question of professional knowledge, and develops a strategy for improving your knowledge base through research awareness.

In the third Section (P4), we consider the nursing profession itself, what it means to be a nurse, and in particular what it means for you as a practitioner to acquire level-2 competences.

The term ends with the first Section of the Management module (M1), which begins to explore your own management role, both as an individual and as a nurse.

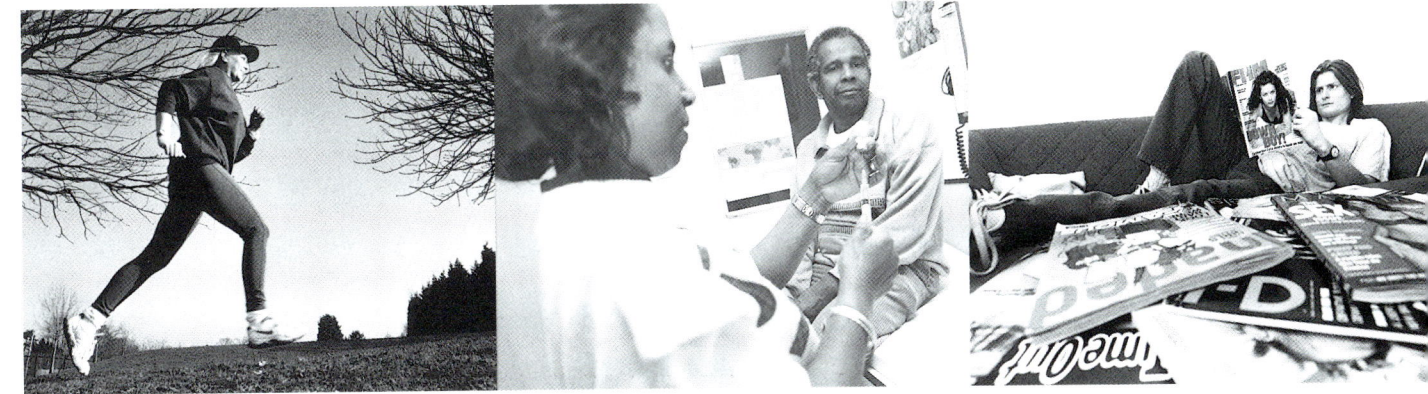

Public health and personal health

How far can we as individuals take responsibility for our health? In this first Part of *P3: Human Environment*, we will discuss the relationship between personal and state responsibility for health.

Here, and in *P3(ii): Organising the nation's health*, you will read some history of the development of public healthcare in this country. This charts the way in which the state began to take more and more responsibility for people's health. For example, 150 years ago water was a significant source of disease and death. Individuals were largely powerless to control this; it needed political action to ensure that water was not contaminated.

You will look at:

- The extent to which we rely on the state to maintain good health

- The Babbage Report of 1850 on 'sewage, drainage and supply of water'

- Different types of statistics and how to use them

- The Public Health Act of 1848 and the Clean Air Act of 1958.

WORK PLANNER

In Activity 6 you will do some simple work on the analysis of statistical tables. You will need the latest edition of *Regional Trends*, published by The Stationery Office. This is available in the reference section of most public libraries. If you feel you need more practice or support, contact your tutor/counsellor.

PERSONAL HEALTH

Most of us believe we have some personal responsibility for our own health, and, increasingly, both the media and the government support this belief. At a basic level, most of us would not wear damp clothes, while some of us jog or swim regularly and are careful about what we eat. However, not all individuals are able to take the same level of responsibility for their own health.

ACTIVITY 1
diary
List the factors you think might affect a person's ability to take responsibility for his or her own health.

FEEDBACK

Whatever actual words you use, most of the items in your list could probably be categorised as 'knowledge', 'attitudes' or 'abilities'.

Notes

ACTIVITY 2
diary
Have another look at the factors you listed in Activity 1 and see if you can group them in that way.

Much of the knowledge we have about looking after our own health at a basic level could be considered 'common-sense' habits which our parents taught us, such as eating all our vegetables. This sort of knowledge is passed on between generations. Other knowledge comes from health promotion sources, which use knowledge based on scientific research, so many people now have more information about the nutritional value of foods. Other examples include having children immunised and always taking a dog out with a 'pooper scooper'.

These sources of knowledge about health will have different levels of importance with different individuals. Some people may prefer to trust the wisdom of knowledge based on generations of experience, rather than 'new' information which is the product of scientific research. However, the point we want to consider here is whether, whatever the source of information on which we base our decisions, we can take full and sole responsibility for our own health.

ACTIVITY 3
discussion
In your view, is it possible, given adequate and accurate information, for an individual to take complete responsibility for his or her own personal health in each of the following areas?:
1. Diet
2. Immunisation
3. Diseases transmitted by dog excreta.

FEEDBACK

A sensible diet requires knowledge of the sorts and amounts of food that are necessary for health, and a positive attitude towards taking heed of that information. It also requires an ability to buy that food. Ensuring that all members of any society have adequate means to buy a healthy diet requires a state-run system of *social security*, which guarantees that no one's income falls below an agreed minimum level.

Immunisation requires both knowledge and acceptance by parents, and a system whereby immunisation is available to every child. That means either that each family must be able to afford to pay for the immunisations or that there is some nationally co-ordinated and funded system for providing it. The *National Health Service* supplies this service in the United Kingdom.

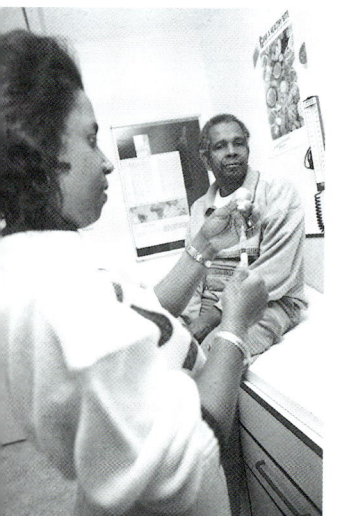

You might try to avoid dog excreta, given that you were fully informed of, and accepted, the dangers of such excrement. However, a much more effective method is to have *laws* that make the fouling of public areas by dogs a legal offence. The prevention of contamination by dog excreta thus becomes the responsibility of the *public health sector*, and the law is used as a means of promoting health.

In the above examples we have three items that could be said to be the health responsibility of individuals but which actually require action on a public level. We shall be looking at Britain's health and social security provision in more detail later on. Here we will concentrate on how legal measures have been used to improve public health in this country.

ACTIVITY 4
diary
Note down any ways in which you think the state takes some responsibility for the nation's health. We shall come back to this Activity later on.

PUBLIC HEALTH

Before we come back to the Activity, it might shed some light on the way things are today if we compare them with the situation 150 years ago.

Evidence from the Past

In 1850, the Revd Patrick Brontë, the father of Emily, author of *Wuthering Heights*, and Charlotte, author of *Jane Eyre*, helped initiate an inquiry into:

'the sewerage, drainage, and supply of water, and the sanitary condition of the inhabitants of the hamlet of Haworth.'

Haworth was the hamlet in West Yorkshire in which the Brontës lived. Mr Brontë's concern for the health of his parishioners arose from the widespread disease he saw around him, and from which his own family had suffered. The report resulting from the inquiry, the *Babbage Report*[1], reached a number of conclusions, which are listed below. Have a look at them now.

The Babbage Report 1850: Summary of the conclusions[1]

1. That the annual mortality of the hamlet of Haworth is 25.4 in the thousand, whilst the mortality of the neighbouring hamlet is only 17.6 in the thousand.

2. That a large pecuniary loss, equivalent to a rate of at least 6s in the pound, falls upon the inhabitants of Haworth in consequence of this excessive mortality.

3. That 41.6 per cent of the people born, die before attaining the age of six years.

4. That the average age at death is 25.8 years, which corresponds with that of some of the most unhealthy of the London districts.

5. That 21.7% of the population die without receiving any medical assistance, and that this fact offers great facilities for the commission of crime.

6. That the number of privies* is unusually small, averaging only one to every four-and-a-half-houses.

7. That no sewerage exists to carry off refuse and decomposing matter, and that the exposed cesspools are very offensive and injurious to health.

8. That the present water supply is extremely limited in quantity, and that in the summer much of it is deleterious in quality.

9. That the parish churchyard is so full of graves that no more interments should be allowed.

10. That an efficient system of sewerage may be laid down at an average weekly charge of $3/4$ d per house, that an ample supply of pure water would cost $1^1/_4$ d per house weekly upon average, and that such of the houses as require it may have water laid on, be properly drained, and have the present offensive privies converted into water closets, at a weekly charge of 1d.

   'Privies' were lavatories where there was no drainage and they were therefore a great health hazard and very foul smelling. Water closets, or 'WCs' as they became known, could have the contents flushed away by water into drainage sewers.

Simple Statistics

Although financial comparisons are difficult because of the changing values of money over the past 150 years, comparisons of death rates, often called 'mortality rates', are not.

Numerical records gathered over time can be classified in a variety of ways to throw light on particular issues or problems, such as the numbers and distribution of people suffering from particular diseases. This gathering and classifying of data is called *statistical analysis*, and it allows, for example, the mapping of the health of a nation or of smaller areas such as health districts. The statistics of one country can be compared with those of another, and of one health authority, or other type of area, with another.

EXAMPLE

It is statistics of this type that have identified the 'clusters' of leukaemia that we now know occur in particular locations, and that have highlighted the occupations of the fathers of children with leukaemia as a possible contributing factor to the children's developing the disease.

The types of statistics that can be used to analyse various aspects of a nation or region's health can be divided up as follows[2]:

Notes

1. Demographic statistics, such as population, marriages and fertility (births)

2. Mortality statistics, such as numbers and causes of death

3. Morbidity statistics, such as illness and injuries, incapacity and hospitalisation.

Such statistics are usually expressed in numbers of the item being counted, such as deaths, for each thousand of population each year. Yearly health statistics are published by the government, together with those on population, education, employment, income, expenditure, housing, transport and law enforcement, in *Social Trends*, which covers national statistics, and in *Regional Trends*, which breaks down the statistical information into regions.

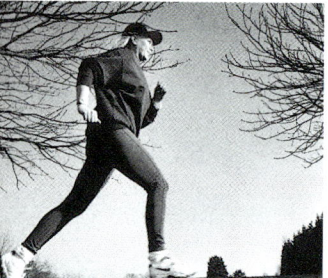

Then and Now

Statistics in the 1850 Babbage report show that the mortality rate for Haworth was a yearly rate of 25.4 per thousand population. This means that each year 25 people in each thousand living in that area would die. Don't worry about the 0.4 – statistics rarely work out to round figures because populations are rarely whole thousands to divide into!

The mortality rate in Haworth at that time, although higher than that in the neighbouring hamlet, was not unusual. The national mortality rate in 1850 exceeded 23 per thousand population. A modern comparison will show how much progress has been made. The details in the table below will allow you to compare the historical mortality rates we have been discussing with more recent ones. You may find it easier to use the table if you photocopy it first.

The table shown below contains a lot of information. The best way to extract this information is to take a step-by-step approach. Read the title of the table and then the list down the left-hand side. You now know that you are going to look at the statistics for health authority areas for 1996. The list down the left-hand side shows that statistics will be printed across the top line from left to right for the whole United Kingdom, and similarly across the table for each of the health authorities areas and the four countries that make up the United Kingdom.

Population and vital statistics: NHS Regional Office areas, 1996[3].

	Population aged (mid-year estimates) (thousands)					Vital statistics (rates)				
	0–15	16–64	65–84	85 or over	All ages	Live births[1]	Still births[2]	Deaths[3]	Perinatal mortality[4]	Infant mortality[5]
United Kingdom	12,098.3	37,452.4	8,183.6	1,067.2	58,801.5	60.1	5.5	10.9	8.7	6.1
Northern and Yorkshire	1,309.6	4,018.8	898.3	111.4	6,338.0	58.7	5.4	11.3	8.6	8.4
North West	1,400.8	4,170.7	915.6	118.0	6,605.1	60.7	5.5	11.6	8.7	6.4
Trent	1,038.5	3,257.3	735.7	89.7	5,121.2	58.5	5.4	10.9	8.7	6.3
West Midlands	1,119.5	3,369.0	741.6	86.5	5,316.6	62.7	6.1	10.6	10.2	6.8
Anglia and Oxford	1,113.3	3,456.4	699.1	92.1	5,360.9	59.2	4.9	9.6	7.7	5.8
North Thames	1,428.1	4,535.1	852.5	118.0	6,933.7	63.4	6.1	9.5	9.0	5.6
South Thames	1,354.4	4,352.9	964.0	147.8	6,819.1	60.8	5.3	10.9	8.6	6.1
South and West	1,288.6	4,124.0	1,032.3	149.5	6,594.4	58.4	4.6	11.3	7.5	5.5
England	10,052.7	31,284.2	6,839.1	913.1	49,089.1	60.4	5.4	10.7	8.6	6.1
Wales	602.0	1,812.4	450.2	56.4	2,921.1	61.1	4.9	11.9	7.5	5.6
Scotland	1,028.0	3,320.6	700.8	78.7	5,128.0	54.0	6.4	11.8	9.2	6.2
Northern Ireland	415.6	1,035.2	193.5	19.0	1,663.3	68.0	6.3	9.1	9.4	5.8

1 Per 1,000 women aged 15–44.

2 Per 1,000 live and still births. A still birth relates to a baby born dead after 24 completed weeks gestation or more.

3 Per 1,000 population.

4 Still births and deaths of infants under 1 week of age per 1,000 live and still births.

5 Deaths of infants under 1 year of age per 1,000 live births.

Source: Office for National Statistics; General Register Office for Scotland; Northern Ireland Statistics and Research Agency

Now look at the layout of the rest of the table (don't worry about individual figures yet). The first four columns which run from top to bottom give numbers of the population, with 'all ages' in the fifth column of figures, which are also broken down, in the preceding four columns, into different age groups, '0–15', '16–64', '65–84', and '85 or over'. The last five columns give the 'vital statistics', that is, those concerned with life and death. The small figures beside each of those headings are explained at the bottom of the chart, so we know that the numbers in the 'Live births' column is for births per 1,000 women aged 15–44, and so on.

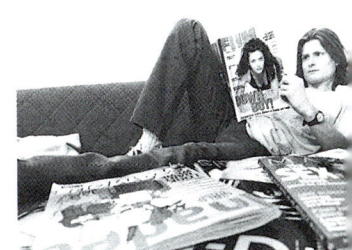

ACTIVITY 5
knowledge base

Have a look at the third column from the right, headed 'Deaths'. The figure 3 beside that heading relates to Note 3 at the bottom of the chart that tells us that these figures are for each 1,000 population. Now note down the death rate given in that column for the United Kingdom, the Northern and Yorkshire health authority area in which Haworth lies, and your own health authority area.

FEEDBACK

The deaths per thousand of population in the United Kingdom are shown as 10.9, and that is the first figure you should have written down. The deaths in Northern and Yorkshire health authority area were 11.3, the second figure in your written list. We can't check your third figure as we don't know your particular health authority area, but if you have not got the same figures for the first two as we have, go back now and find the places from which we took them. Then do Activity 5 again to make sure you are clear about it.

ACTIVITY 6
knowledge base

Find a copy of the latest edition of *Regional Trends*, published by The Stationery Office. Don't be alarmed at the large numbers of charts and figures in it. The example you have just been working through came from an earlier edition, so you now know you can cope with it. Browse through it from beginning to end, finding out what each chart or graph shows, but without worrying too much about individual figures. This will give you an idea of the sort of information you can find in it, and similar publications, should you need to do so in the future. Then find the chart for population and vital statistics in the section on health. Note down the mortality rate for your health authority area and compare it with the national average.

Why was the mortality rate in 1850 so high compared with the rate today, and why are there still variations from one part of the country to another? The second question is considered in *P7: Health Promotion.* Our task here is to look at the great advances that were made in public health because of the work and ideas of a succession of people with imagination, compassion and practical natures — people who saw problems, analysed them and thought out workable solutions.

PUBLIC HEALTH LAWS

Perhaps the greatest character of 19th-century public health reform was Edwin Chadwick, a Member of Parliament with a social conscience. Chadwick was convinced that health depended on a system of sanitation, in which the incoming water supplies and the outgoing sewage and other contaminated materials were kept totally separate. This would also mean the control of contaminants placed in the ground, which in those days included almost all dead bodies. In Haworth in the 10 years prior to 1850, there had been 1,344 burials in a churchyard of less than one acre, with no adequate drainage; inevitably, the drainage from the graveyard must have contaminated water collected from wells lower down the hill.

Chadwick's *Public Health Act of 1848* was the first public health Act. In truth, this Act had very little scientific basis because there was no actual proof of the bacterial origins of much of the disease from which the population suffered. Nevertheless, it was a landmark in the history of public health[4].

The Public Health Act 1848 led to a 'sanitary revolution' by creating a body of skilled public health experts[5]. The main provisions of this Act were to set up local boards of health which would appoint a surveyor, inspector of nuisances, treasurer and clerk, and an officer of health who had to be a legally qualified medical practitioner. The local board of health was required to keep all sewers in a manner such that they would not be a health hazard. It became unlawful to build any house without drains or without an adequate 'water closet, privy or ashpit'[6].

There had to be provision for all streets, including pavements, to be properly swept, cleansed and watered. The boards might also, if they thought fit, provide sanitary conveniences for the public — the first public lavatories.

Mr Brontë and his colleagues used the 1848 Act to empower the setting up of the Haworth Inquiry. The main recommendations of the resulting Babbage Report[1] were that:

- Glazed earthenware sewers be laid down, and that the sewage be distributed for manure

- A public slaughtering house be established

- All cesspools be abolished, that a supply of water be brought into each house, and that at least one properly constructed water closet be made for every three houses

- An ample supply of water be brought to Hawarth and distributed through branch mains and service pipes

- No future interments be allowed in the present parish churchyard and that a code of rules be made to regulate all future interments, whether burial grounds or cemeteries

- All future interments in vaults be prohibited.

So successful was this report that, when Mr Brontë died in 1861, special permission had to be obtained to allow his burial in the family vault in Haworth church.

ACTIVITY 7
diary
Look back at Activity 4. Did you include in your list responsibility for your water supply, sewage disposal and the disposal of bodies?

In answering Activity 4, you might also have included a number of other items such as unpolluted air and the accumulation of rubbish.

The Clean Air Act 1958 controlled the atmospheric pollution that was then causing terrible respiratory problems, particularly in heavily built-up and industrial areas. This Act initiated 'smoke control areas' in which it is prohibited to emit smoke from a chimney — the so-called 'smoke-free zones'.

There is now a vast amount of legislation concerned with public action on the health of the nation generally, and some of it is the reason why the national mortality rate is no longer 25 per thousand.

Did you also include in your answer to Activity 4 the measures taken by the state to promote healthy behaviour in individuals — such as encouraging healthy eating and highlighting the dangers of cigarette smoking, alcohol and drug abuse?

To conclude this discussion on public health legislation, we would like you to reflect on some of the issues surrounding any laws to control threats to individual and public health.

ACTIVITY 8
discussion
Consider action already taken to control the effects of cigarette smoking on public health. Do you think the state should take more responsibility than it already does for reducing this threat? What factors could limit the amount of responsibility the state might be prepared to accept?

What Now?

By now you may well have asked: 'What about the greenhouse effect, the pollution of food, or the contamination of water from industrial waste buried in the ground?' As our technology has advanced, it seems that our respect for our environment has lessened as we have bombarded our planet with air-borne, water-borne and buried poisons. Since we breathe in air, grow food in the ground and cannot live without water, we must surely now take urgent action. What we as individuals can do to protect ourselves from these dangers to our health is limited. Our personal health depends upon public health policy and action.

FOCUS

Consider one or more of your social or nursing client groups. Think about aspects of the health of that group of individuals. Identify:

- Those aspects for which the individual has responsibility

- Those for which there is public responsibility

- Those where there is an overlapping of responsibilities between the two.

For example, in the case of sanitation in the home, the individual has a responsibility to ensure that sewage is discharged into drains. The Public Health Department has a responsibility to maintain good drainage and deal with disposal of the sewage. In this case there is an overlap between individual and public responsibility.

REFERENCES

1   Babbage, H. *Babbage Report*. London: HMSO, 1850.
2   Logan W.P.D., Lambert P.M. Vital statistics. In: Hobson. W. *The Theory and Practice of Public Health*. London: Oxford University Press, 1975.
3   *Regional Trends* 33. London: The Stationery Office, 1998.
4   Fraser-Brockington C. The history of public health. In: Hobson, W. *The Theory and Practice of Public Health*. London: Oxford University Press, 1975.
5   Frazer, W.M. *A History of English Public Health*. London: Bailliere, Tindall & Cox, 1950.
6   *Public Health Act 1848*, Section 49. London: HMSO, 1848.

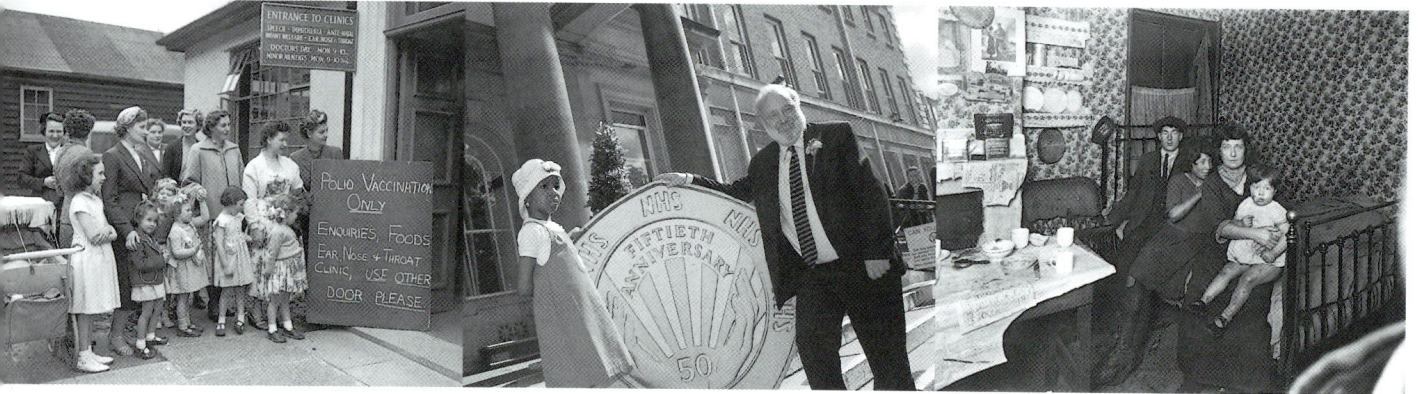

Notes

Organising the nation's health

This Part looks at how state support for health has developed and is now provided in Britain. It does not give you a complete historical account; but some of the history leading up to the establishment of the welfare state gives an important perspective on how far we have come and how far we could still go.

In this Part we will tell you about:

- The Beveridge Report

- The key components of the welfare state

- Social security and social services today

- Change in the National Health Service.

WORK PLANNER

In Activity 2 you are asked to interview someone over the age of 75 if possible. You should plan your interview carefully, making sure you ask the person's permission. Remember that there are notes on preparing for interviews in your student support packs.

Activity 5 suggests that you update the information you have on social security benefits available to the people in your care. Schedule some time to call into your local social security office to pick up some literature

The following books are essential reading for this Part:

- The government White Papers *Working for Patients* (1989, Cmnd 555, HMSO); *Caring for People* (1989, Cmnd 849, HMSO); *The New NHS: Modern, Dependable* (1997, Cmnd 3807, The Stationery Office)

- Helen Forrester's *Twopence to Cross the Mersey* (William Collins Sons & Co. Ltd, 1986)

- Audrey Leathard's *Health Care Provision, Past, Present and Future* (Chapman and Hall, 1990).

SOCIAL WELFARE

P3(i): Public health and personal health looked back to a time when there was no public health policy in Britain, and when people died in their thousands because of a contaminated water supply and lack of efficient disposal of sewage and refuse. The progress that was made in public health after the passing of the first Public Health Act in 1848 gave some positive health benefits to most members of society. However, poverty persisted, and inadequate housing, nutrition, education, employment and income continued as social scourges. In her biography of her childhood in Liverpool in the 1930s, Helen Forrester[1] describes the terrible conditions in which her family lived:

'Only years later, when I saw pictures of the prisoners released from Belsen, did I fully realise how close we were to dying of starvation, and also what an ordeal it must have been for those children at school to drag themselves there and back and try to pay attention while their bodies gradually wasted'.

Social problems can range from the starvation described by Helen Forrester and the inadequate housing and unemployment that the family also endured, to lack of access to health promotion and facilities because of language and cultural differences.

ACTIVITY 1
diary
Note down any health and social problems that you have observed in our present society that you don't think are being adequately dealt with at present. We come back to your answers in Activity 3.

THE BEVERIDGE REPORT

The Second World War caused the health of the nation to become a focus of public concern. A country cannot fight wars with a weak and unhealthy population! However, apart from this pressing need, there were those with genuine social consciences who worried about the suffering among many members of the population that had little to do with the war. Most notable among these was William Beveridge, chairman of a committee whose recommendations in the *Beveridge Report*[2], published in 1942, were the foundation of the welfare state in Great Britain.

The *Beveridge Report* set out three basic assumptions for adequate social provision, which we quote here:

A: Children's Allowances

'That there should be a general scheme of children's allowances in which direct provision for the maintenance of dependent children would be made by payment of allowances to those responsible for the care of those children.'

This was the idea behind the payment of a 'family allowance', now known as 'child benefit'.

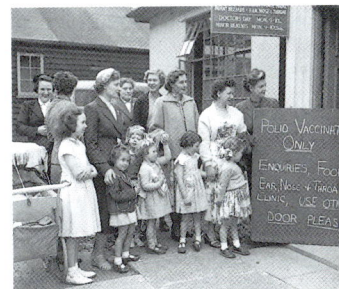

B: Comprehensive Health and Rehabilitation Services

'The second of the three assumptions has two sides to it. It covers a national health service for prevention and for cure of disease and disability by medical treatment; it covers rehabilitation and fitting for employment by treatment which will be both medical and post-medical.'

This assumption recommended a comprehensive national health service that would ensure:

'That for every citizen there is available whatever medical treatment he requires, in whatever form he requires it, domiciliary or institutional, general specialist or consultant, and ... the provision of dental, ophthalmic and surgical appliances, nursing and midwifery and rehabilitation after accidents.'

This was the inspiration for the creation of the National Health Service.

C: Maintenance of Employment

This assumption was based on the belief that:

'The state of the labour market has a direct bearing on rehabilitation and recovery of injured and sick persons and upon the possibility of giving to those suffering from partial infirmities, such as deafness, the chance of a happy and useful career.'

In *P1(i) A personal view of health and illness* we referred to Albert, whose refusal to have his ischaemic leg amputated was based on the pity and contempt in which 'cripples' were held. Until the *Beveridge Report*, the employment of people with disabilities was virtually unheard of and they were seen as an unrelieved burden on their families.

The plan under this assumption was for:

'A scheme of social insurance against interruption and destruction of earning power and for special expenditure arising at birth, marriage or death ... to make want under any circumstances unnecessary.'

This was the foundation of the social security system.

ACTIVITY 2
action
Ask at least one person over 75, if possible, to talk to you about his or her opinions on the introduction of child allowances and the National Health Service. Ask for the person's experiences and opinions on the problems of unemployment before the war. It may help to take a tape recorder along so that you can, with the permission of the person you are interviewing, share his or her recollections and opinions with your colleagues.

The five giant evils: Towards the end of the report, Beveridge makes this comment:

'There are some who will say that pursuit of security as defined in this Report, that is to say income security, is a wholly inadequate aim. The Plan for Social Security is put forward as part of a general programme of social policy. It is one part only of an attack upon five giant evils: upon the *want* with which it is directly concerned; upon *disease*, which often causes that want and brings many other troubles in its train; upon *ignorance* which no democracy can afford amongst its citizens; upon the *squalor* which arises mainly through haphazard distribution of industry and population; and upon the *idleness* which destroys wealth and corrupts men, whether they are well fed or not, when they are idle.'

ACTIVITY 3
diary
Look back at the problems you listed in Activity 1. Can you group them under the headings of the five giant evils identified by Beveridge: want, disease, ignorance, squalor and idleness? For example, if you put down 'unfit population' you could list that under both 'want', because it might be due to an inadequate diet resulting from an inadequate income, and under 'ignorance' because it might also be connected to obesity from poor eating habits.

THE WELFARE STATE

When the welfare state came into being in Britain following the election of a socialist government in the first general election after the end of the Second World War, it was a virtual social revolution. Although the welfare state did not include all the innovations that Beveridge had wanted, it did make tremendous strides towards providing a decent standard of living and health care for the population.

The National Insurance Act 1946: The new welfare state provided the first true system of 'social security' in this country. It provided for unemployment benefit, retirement pension, widow's benefit, guardians' allowance and death grant being paid to those covered by National Insurance contributions. This scheme fell short of Beveridge's proposals but it did remove much extreme poverty and was the first part of the giant stride of social progress that was to take place.

Housing: The beliefs which had brought about the welfare state also provided the impetus for major programmes of house-building by local authorities. At the end of the war there were 700,000 fewer houses than there had been when it started and in the three years after the war there were 33% more births than there had been in the three years before it[3]. There is now considerable evidence that there is a strong link between health and housing[4], and the overcrowding that resulted from the post-war housing shortage must have taken its toll in both physical and mental illness.

In 1996, there were 1,079,610 homeless households and in 1997 there were 1,065,790 — a small decrease[5].

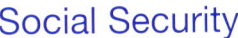

**ACTIVITY 4
diary**
Can you identify any possible links between housing and health today? Make a note of the groups of people most affected.

The National Health Service Act 1946: The opening sentences of the National Health Service Act set out its aims of providing a comprehensive health service designed to secure improvement in the physical and mental health of the people of England and Wales. The health service was to prevent, diagnose and treat illness and was to be free at the point of delivery. However, we must bear in mind, as we saw in previous discussions on funding health care, that the money has to come from somewhere even though the individual does not pay when receiving care.

Although there was much opposition from doctors, the National Health Service came into being as had been planned, completing the giant stride forward in social progress in post-war Britain.

THE STATE AND HEALTH TODAY

The 1946 Act laid the foundation for today's provision, but there have been many changes in the half-century since the welfare state first came into being in this country. The British social welfare system now comprises

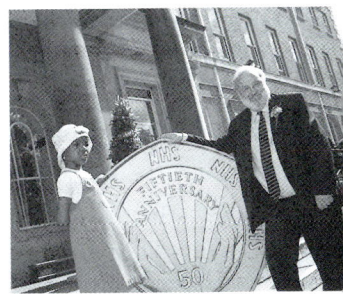

- The social security and personal social services.

- The National Health Service.

Social Security

The stated aim of the present social security programme is to 'provide an efficient and responsive system of financial help for people who are elderly, sick, disabled, unemployed, widowed or bringing up children'[6]. There is said to be provision for people who have 'insufficient means of support'.

**ACTIVITY 5
action**
Are you familiar with the range of social security provision for your clients or patients? You may want to get hold of some up-to-date literature so that you can pass information on to the people in your care when the need arises.

Reflect on community care for families living in 'bed and breakfast' accommodation paid for by local authorities. These families experience both mental and physical stress from this situation. Toilet and cooking facilities are often inadequate for the numbers of people who have to prepare food for themselves in overcrowded rooms with few facilities to do so, or for children to play safely.

The Changing National Health Service

The NHS is now Europe's biggest organisation:

'It has a workforce of around one million people who provide care and treatment for many millions more every year. The NHS spends in excess of £42 billion — the largest item of central government expenditure after social security'[7].

In 1998 the NHS website described the purpose of the NHS as being to:

'secure through the resources available the greatest possible improvement in the physical and mental health of the nation by: promoting health, preventing ill-health, diagnosing and treating injury and disease and caring for those with long-term illness and disability who require the service of the NHS'[8].

ACTIVITY 6
diary
Compare the definition of the purpose of the NHS given at the bottom of the previous page with that given in the *Beveridge Report* in 1942, outlined on page 69.

As a public service funded by the taxpayer, the NHS is accountable to the government and to Parliament. Different arrangements exist in different parts of the UK — both in governmental responsibilities for the NHS and how those responsibilities are discharged. Your local library should be able to give you access to information on different arrangements.

At present, just over 80% of the cost of the health service in Britain is paid for by general taxation; the rest is met from the National Health Service contribution paid with the National Insurance contribution and from charges towards such items as drugs. In addition, our tax has to cover central government, the security of the nation — both internal, by contributing to the cost of the police service, and external, by helping finance the armed services — some transport resources, such as major trunk road projects, and social security and pensions.

ACTIVITY 7
diary
Do you think you pay too much, about the right amount or too little tax? What services or items would you be prepared to pay more or less for?

If you find these issues interesting, a browse through the latest copy of *Britain 1998: An official handbook*[6] will give you further information on how your tax and National Insurance contributions are used.

ACTION NOW

We live in a democracy, in which there is government by the people through their elected representatives in Parliament and on local councils. How does our democracy deal with the problems of health which inadequate levels of social provision may foster?

The *Beveridge Report* had this comment towards its end:

'Freedom from want cannot be forced on a democracy or given to a democracy. It must be won by them. Winning it needs courage and faith and a sense of national unity; courage to face facts and difficulties and overcome them; faith in our future and in the ideas of fair play and freedom for which century after century our forefathers were prepared to die; a sense of national unity overriding the interests of any class or nation.'

ACTIVITY 8
diary
Describe your own feelings on the ways in which our society is dealing at present with the problems you listed in Activity 3, under Beveridge's 'five giant evils'. What action do you think the government should take to overcome these problems?

The Labour government has recognised the link between health, welfare and housing. The Health Improvement Initiative, together with the establishment of Health Action Zones, are seen as providing a framework for organisations from each of these sectors to work together to overcome deprivation and hardship. Health Action Zones, in particular, are expected to address the public health needs of a local area as well as speeding up the response of health services.

What do you do at present to try and improve health in society as a whole, apart from working as a nurse? For example, did you vote in all the elections in which you were eligible to do so, general, local council or professional? Do you attend meetings where health problems are on the agenda and contribute to the discussions where appropriate?

ACTIVITY 9
diary
Note down any action you have taken in the past 12 months, apart from actually working as a nurse, that could be described as making a positive contribution to health care.

In *P1(iii): Professionals and consumers* the notion of nurses using their professional status to give authority to their opinion on any subject under discussion was considered. The possible pitfalls of this 'Well, as a nurse I think that ...' approach were discussed. But what about the other side of that coin? Are there any benefits to using well-informed, rational and co-ordinated professional opinion to bring about change?

The nursing profession is a very large group and its size should give its members power in any healthcare decision-making process. Why, then, are nurses often ignored by those in power, both at local and national levels?

ACTIVITY 10
discussion
Consider whether you think the nursing profession generally fails to get its voice heard. Make a note of your thoughts in your diary and discuss your view with colleagues or in your own study group.

FEEDBACK

There are many possible views. You might have said that we are a mainly female profession in a society that is still dominated by a male-centred culture. Are we still too used to giving way to the power of mainly male groups? It is also possible that we still do not really respect ourselves as a fully fledged profession with a totally credible knowledge, skills and experience base from which to argue in any health debate. As a group we possibly still do not believe that our opinions are as worthy of note as those of the mainly male and more securely established medical profession.

However, perhaps the most important factor is that we are not sufficiently well organised to bring about change.

ACTIVITY 11
diary
When did you last attend a professional meeting (other than one connected with pay negotiations)? What subject was discussed?

Although we all recognise that concerted action on pay is vital if we are to attract the right quality of people into our profession, and keep them in it, there are many broad social problems related to health that we ought also to be involved in fighting, some of which we have been discussing in this Part. Have your actions so far been adequate? What more could you do?

NURSES AND POLITICS

Many of us think that being 'political' means being on one political 'wing' or the other. It may very well be true for some people, but it is perfectly possible to have strong political feelings without being either totally to the 'right', to the 'left', 'middle of the road' or 'green'. For example you may agree with the social welfare policies of the socialist left and with the general environmental policies of the Green party, but disagree strongly with the disarmament policies of both of them. You may agree strongly with the education policies of the political right but disagree with their plans for the reorganisation of the health service.

To be politically minded and to take political action does not mean that you necessarily have to belong to any particular political group. It does mean that you gather and consider facts and proposals and discuss them with others, which is quite different from expressing an ill-considered and undebated viewpoint. It should follow that you enter into professional debate and increase the voice and power of nurses as a credible professional group.

Bear in mind that some of your professional journals are political. Consider the *Nursing Times* mission statement:

'*Nursing Times* is the independent voice of nursing. It is radical, challenging and professional and aims to inform, inspire and entertain. It campaigns for a better deal for patients and for the nurses, midwives and health visitors who care for them'[9].

Democracy gives power to the people. Nurses are a group within a democracy, and it is time that we organised ourselves more efficiently so that we can use our portion of democratic power to some effect.

We hope you have enjoyed considering these very important and quite difficult areas of debate. We have moved a long way from William Beveridge but not far enough from the giant evils he brought to public awareness. What happens now is the choice of all members of our democracy. Make sure that you play your part.

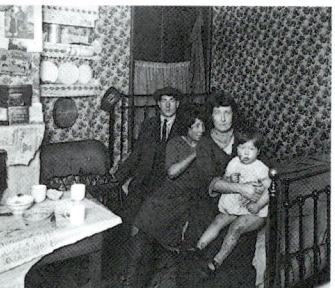

FOCUS

Read the White Paper *The New NHS: Modern, Dependable*[10]. Consider the healthcare problems you noted in your answer to Activity 1. Do you think the White Paper helps or hinders the solution of these problems?

Prepare a short report (two pages) using each of the healthcare problems you noted in Activity 1 as headings.

REFERENCES

1   Forrester H. *Twopence to Cross the Mersey.* Glasgow: William Collins Sons & Co. Ltd., 1986.
2   Beveridge, Lord. *The Beveridge Report in Brief.* London: HMSO, 1942.
3   Sked A., Cook C. *Post-war Britain.* Harmondsworth: Penguin Books Ltd., 1979.
4   Conway, J. (ed). *Prescription for Poor Health. The crisis for homeless families.* London: London Food Commission, The Maternity Alliance, SHAC and Shelter, 1988.
5   *Social Trends 20.* London: HMSO, 1998.
6   *Britain 1998: An official handbook.* London: Her Majesty's Stationery Office, 1998.
7   www.nhs50.uk/nhstoday-understand-index,htm 1998.
8   www.nhs50.uk/nhstoday-understand-index,htm nhs 1998.
9   *Nursing Times.* Mission Statement. *Nursing Times* 1997; **93**: 6, 3.
10 Department of Health. *The New NHS: Modern, Dependable.* London: The Stationery Office, Cmnd 3807, 1997.

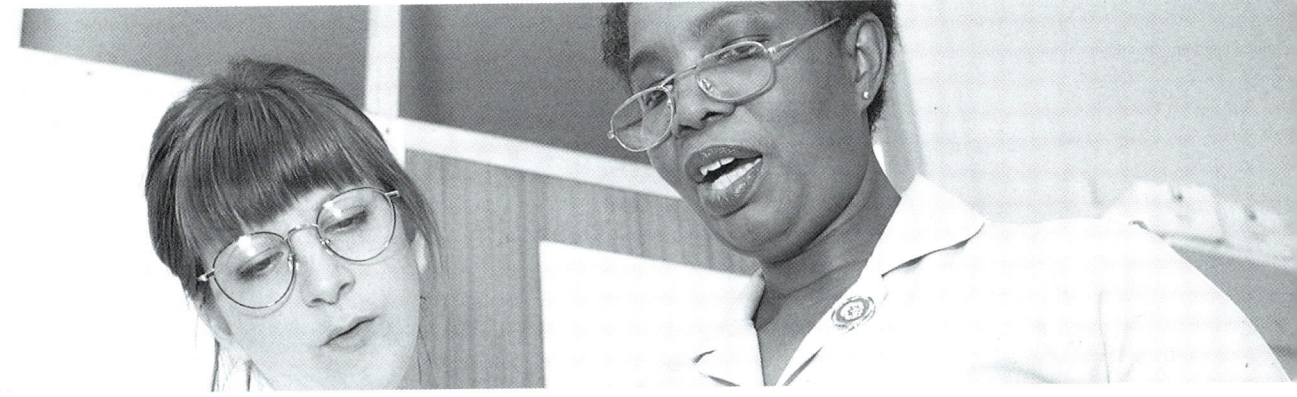

Sources of knowledge

In this Part you make a systematic plan to increase and enhance your knowledge. You will look at:

- Where knowledge comes from in everyday life
- The sources of knowledge used in nursing practice
- Why we need to expand our nursing knowledge
- How to identify 'good quality' knowledge
- Learning from experience.

WORK PLANNER

Activities 7, 8 and 9 will take up to 1 hour to complete, so you may want to do some careful time-planning.

You will need to have a book on nursing practice at hand to complete Activity 7 and a copy of *Nursing Times* to complete Activity 8.

You are asked to have a discussion with a friend or colleague in Activities 5 and 9.

For Activity 10 you will need to make an arrangement to spend half-a-day in a nursing area you have never been to before.

EXPLORING YOUR KNOWLEDGE RESOURCES

We all know where personal, or experiential, knowledge comes from: it results from all the varied experiences which we have in life. But we do not learn everything from experience. There are other ways in which we acquire knowledge. In everyday life we pick up new pieces of information all the time — news items, new recipes, information about our partner's work or our children's school work. We get this information or knowledge from a variety of sources. Books are one *medium* or *channel* from which we gain our knowledge and there are many others.

ACTIVITY 1
diary
Make a list of all the different channels or media through which you learn in your everyday life, that is, channels not specifically related to nursing. You will be using your list as the basis of later Activities.

We started with books, but your list might also have included TV, radio, newspapers, magazines, videos, journals and the Internet.

We also learn from people with whom we are in direct contact.

Notes

ACTIVITY 2
diary
Make a list of all the groups of people with whom you are in direct contact and from whom you learn, for example, friends. Again, think of your life in general rather than specifically nursing.

FEEDBACK

Here is one person's list:

- Evening class teacher
- Partner
- Manager
- Friend
- Children
- Colleagues.

Moving into nursing

You now have a picture of the sources of knowledge in your everyday life: there are the channels or media you identified along with the people who give you pieces of information, while in your nursing practice you also turn to magazines, journals, and videos to gain knowledge. You also learn from colleagues at work.

ACTIVITY 3
diary
Make a list of the sources of knowledge you used for your nursing practice last week. Include people as well as other media. Note down any other sources of knowledge which are important to your nursing practice and which you did not use during the past week.

FEEDBACK

Your list of sources of specifically nursing knowledge might have included procedure, policy or standards documents; nursing journals and, possibly, videos.

The people from whom you gained information might have included nurse teachers or a specialist nurse. We consult specialists because of the knowledge or experience they have of a particular area of care. For example, you might consult a stoma care nurse because she has seen a lot more people with stomas than you have and has a lot of 'tips of the trade' which you would find useful.

EXPANDING YOUR KNOWLEDGE BASE

Having thought about where you go to obtain knowledge in your current practice, we now look at the reasons why we seek new knowledge.

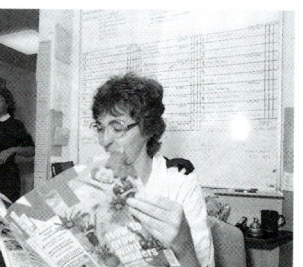

ACTIVITY 4
diary
Think about the occasions during the past week when you felt it would have been useful to amend or enhance your knowledge. Why did this happen? Why was your current knowledge not good enough?

FEEDBACK

There are many reasons why we might seek out new knowledge. Perhaps the most straightforward is when we find ourselves in a situation which we have never encountered before. Our existing knowledge in such an instance is insufficient and we have to find a way of dealing with the problem.

One example might be a new area of work, or having a patient admitted with a problem that you have never had to deal with before.

Gaps in your knowledge could also be highlighted by someone asking you a question which you find difficult to answer properly; for example:

- 'Why do I have to starve from midnight?'
- 'If I do take the blue pills before the red pills, what will happen?'
- 'The other nurse said I have to sleep with my arm raised; why do you say I don't?'

Colleagues, relatives, clients and general managers can all ask us questions which we cannot answer.

Another reason why you might want to seek out new knowledge is because you realise — perhaps through feedback from clients or relatives — that your nursing care is not reaching the standard which you set for yourself, or which you have agreed with your colleagues in a formal standard. You know that you need to improve the care you give but you're not sure how.

All these examples involve situations where the questions are generated through your practice. But the questions might come from a source outside your practice. You might read or hear something which recommends doing things a different way. For example, you might have read an article advocating primary nursing, and while you are not immediately convinced, you think: 'I need to find out more about this.'

EVIDENCE-BASED PRACTICE

R1: Nursing: A Research-based Profession introduced the basics of evidence-based practice. In essence, it involves systematically reviewing our current practice, and new initiatives, in the light of existing evidence.

Professional practice should be based on making effective use of the best evidence available when making decisions about individual patients or the delivery of healthcare. Current 'best' evidence means having up-to-date knowledge and information from relevant, valid research about the effects of different forms of healthcare (see 'Hierarchy of Evidence', below). This, in turn, means that healthcare professionals need to evaluate what is:

- Achievable

- Affordable

- Reliable

- Responsive to change.

Evidence-based practice is also based on principles of supporting patients to enable them to become more involved in their care. Part of the ethos of holistic care means finding ways of enabling patients to understand the effect any changes in their care will have on themselves and their families.

In *Evidence-based Healthcare*[1] the author explains that in evidence-based practice, the effectiveness of a service or intervention is measured in terms of achievement of aims and objectives, that is, whether it works. If you have a number of effective interventions, you would then determine which one works in the most effective manner. Or, to put it more simply, effectiveness is the degree to which the desired outcomes are achieved.

Hierarchy of Evidence

Clinical effectiveness is part of the toolkit of evidence-based practice, and involves monitoring, evaluating and changing clinical practice to produce worthwhile benefits. New initiatives and current practice always need to be reviewed in the light of existing evidence.

Muir Gray[1] explains that evidence should be seen as a hierarchy — number 1 in the hierarchy being the strongest sort of evidence, followed by four other criteria:

1. Strong evidence from at least one systematic review of multiple, well-designed randomised controlled trials

2. Strong evidence from at least one properly designed randomised controlled trial of appropriate size

3. Evidence from well-designed trials without randomisation, single group pre-post, cohort, time series or matched case control

4. Evidence from well designed non-experimental studies from more than one centre or research group

5. Opinions of respected authorities, based on clinical evidence, descriptive studies or reports of expert communities.

How to carry out evidence-based practice

To carry out evidence-based practice in nursing you need an understanding of the methodologies:

- Appraising existing evidence

- Carrying out primary research

- Writing clinical guidelines/protocols.

Carrying out evidence-based practice also requires knowledge of clinical audit and other qualitative and quantitative methods. It uses a mixture of knowledge and skills:

- Awareness of the need for evaluation, and identification of appropriate questions

- Literature searching skills

- Critical appraisal skills

- Change management skills.

ACTIVITY 5
discussion
Discuss evidence-based practice with two or three colleagues. Find out what they know about it and how they put it into practice. Ask them for specific examples. If there seem to be conflicting views about it or difficulties understanding it, speak with your tutor on this programme. Make sure you are clear about evidence-based practice and how to apply it in your setting. It is an important strategy in nursing today. Arrange to read one or two of the sources on evidence-based practice listed at the end of this Part.

QUALITY CONTROL

Enhancing your knowledge base is very important to your nursing practice; so it is important that the quality of knowledge which you acquire is good. We know what we mean by 'good quality carpet' or 'good quality vegetables', but what do we mean by 'good quality knowledge'?

ACTIVITY 6
knowledge base
How would you define 'good quality' knowledge? Write a list of words which would help to define 'good quality'.

FEEDBACK

'Good quality' knowledge has all of the following attributes. It is:

- Reliable
- Up-to-date
- Relevant

- Understandable
- Sensible
- Applicable to your situation.

Your difficulty as you use an increasing number of different sources of knowledge is to judge which are reliable and whether you should accept or reject what they are telling you. Let's consider some examples.

A Book

Take a book which you might find to hand such as Wright's *Building and Using a Model of Nursing*[2]. This includes an introduction which indicates the setting in which the author developed his ideas:

'The slow process of change that began in Tameside's Care of the Elderly Unit in 1981 saw an explosion of innovation in the latter part of 1986. This was the year that much of the earlier work came to fruition.'

This clearly sets the ideas in the book in time and space and allows the readers to judge whether they are relevant to them. However, not all the contents of the book come within the framework of that introduction. For example, on page 20 we find the comment:

'Nursing has a special role to play in helping the person.'

Is this a universal truth, the author's opinion, or knowledge derived specifically from the experience at Tameside? We are not told. So even within a book which clearly sets out the foundations of the knowledge it offers, the reader needs to be vigilant about the type of knowledge being given, on a page-by-page basis.

There are other considerations, too. For example:

- When was the book published?

- How up-to-date is it?

- Is a later edition available?

The place of publication is also important: for example, not all books published in the United States will contain information which is relevant to readers in Britain, and vice versa.

ACTIVITY 7
knowledge base
Choose one book on nursing practice which you have used before, either as part of your work on this programme or for another reason. Make some notes on the following:
• What type of knowledge is being offered? Is it based on the authors' experience? Have they summarised the research? Is it based on an idea they have had?
• What is the authors' experience of the subject? Does it make the book a reliable source of knowledge for you on some/all aspects of the subject?
• When was the book written? Does it need to be up to date, or is the message of the book valuable whenever it is read?

For any one topic, you are likely to come across a wide range of different types of source material in books.

EXAMPLE

A list of books relevant to the topic of care of the dying would include the following types:

- Textbooks

- Expert statements — statements about practice by one person (for example, a specialist nurse) or by a group, committee or organisation

- Reviews of the literature

- Ethical/legal commentaries — particularly important in care of the dying

- Patients' or relatives' accounts

- Novels

- Research.

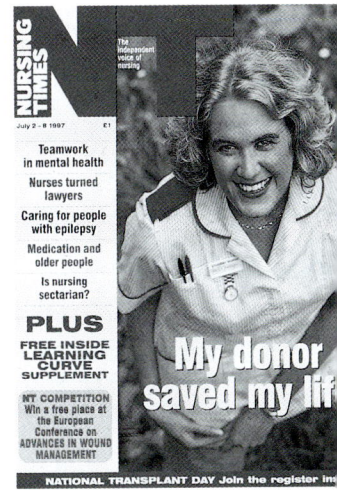

A Nursing Journal

Journals such as *Nursing Times* include a variety of different types of material, such as research reports, letters from readers, commissioned articles on specific topics, and so on. These are all based on different types of knowledge.

The Letters page in particular includes many different types of knowledge. For example, one selection of letters includes the following statements:

'The facts [of a particular situation] are ...'
(presumably the writer is claiming this is research-based knowledge but unfortunately she doesn't include any references.)

'Here in West Scotland we feel ...'
(Is she expressing the mutual knowledge of her group? Has she conducted a scientific survey?)

'I'm pretty fed up with nursing ...'
(This is probably based on her own experience.)

ACTIVITY 8
knowledge base
1. Turn to the Letters page of this week's *Nursing Times* or any other 'general interest' nursing journal. Read each of the letters carefully and try to identify the basis of any information which they give.
2. Find a news or features article in the same journal which interests you and do the same thing.
3. Find a research article (or one which includes an account of research) and try again to identify the basis of the knowledge offered.

You may find that it is not always easy to identify the knowledge base of the material you read. In general, people are really very careless about defining the source of the knowledge they offer other people. In Activity 8, you probably found that the research article made it much clearer how that knowledge was produced.

In this Part of *R2: Focusing on Research Knowledge* we have considered methods of 'quality controlling' our knowledge resources network to ensure that the information we use is 'good'. We return to this notion many times in the rest of the Research module, but we suggest that from now on you apply the methods just discussed to all your sources of new knowledge.

To end this Part we return to the idea of the first paragraph — learning from your own experience — and consider ways in which you can enhance this learning systematically and consciously.

LEARNING FROM EXPERIENCE

First, you can learn a lot from being there and *thinking about* what you experience. This type of learning is an increasingly important part of nursing knowledge, and one which we value greatly on this programme. As a means of emphasising the 'active' nature of the learning process it is sometimes known as *reflection* rather than learning from experience.

Reflection is the process of reviewing an experience of practice in order to describe, analyse, evaluate and so inform learning about practice.

The idea of reflection was developed by many authors; probably the best known in nursing is Schon[3,4]. By looking at how architects and other professional workers learn, he found that much of their knowledge was derived from thinking about the various difficulties they had encountered in practice and considering how they could have tackled them better.

ACTIVITY 9
discussion
Consider a new experience you have had recently either at work or in private life. Spend some time thinking about all aspects of it — perhaps writing a brief note about what happened.
Then choose a friend or colleague and discuss it with him or her, trying to explain clearly what happened and what conclusions you drew from the experience.

The second way in which we can learn from experience is by looking at familiar things differently, as if we were a stranger going into a new situation. Strangers do not have the mutual knowledge of the group to explain everything they see, so they have to think some things through for themselves. Thinking about new events and experiences often causes you to see familiar things in a new light.

Notes

ACTIVITY 10
action

Spend half-a-day in a nursing area which you have never been to before. Try to act like a 'Martian' — take a critical attitude to what you see, and make notes of those things which you find strange. Ask the 'natives' why they are doing things and see if you think their reasons are good enough. If you choose a ward, for example, you might see that one group is often in bed and another group is always rushing about. Ask why this is so (ask the nurses rather than the patients). If you visit the community you might ask the nurses why they spend so much time knocking on doors and finding no one at home.
Did your experience during this Activity change the way you view anything in your own practice?

This Part of *R2: Focusing on Research Knowledge* has looked at your 'resource network' — the pattern of sources of knowledge which you use in practice. It is important that you use this network systematically and with a conscious knowledge of the different types of knowledge that it offers.

In *R2(ii): Rubbing shoulders with research* we look at ways in which you can become more familiar with research-based knowledge. Much of the work will involve using library facilities, so you should plan your time so that you spend at least 6–8 hours working in a library.

FOCUS

Choose a topic in which you are interested; make it reasonably broad, such as 'pain' or 'stress'. List the sources of your knowledge on this subject. Are all the different types of sources discussed in this Part represented? If not, try to find examples of sources which relate to your chosen topic.

Are your record cards of written sources on this subject up-to-date? Do they indicate the type of knowledge offered? If not, spend some time putting your records in order

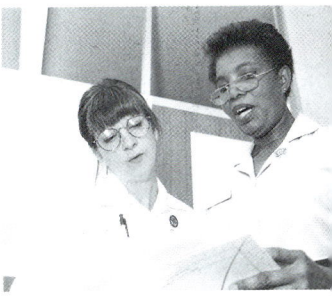

REFERENCES

1   Muir, Gray, J.A. *Evidence-based Healthcare*. London: Churchill Livingstone, 1997.

2   Wright, S. *Building and Using a Model of Nursing*. London: Edward Arnold, 1990.

3   Schon, D. A. *The Reflective Practitioner: How professionals think in action*. London: Temple Smith, 1983.

4   Schon, D. A. *Educating the Reflective Practitioner: Toward a new design for teaching and learning*. London: Jossey Bass, 1987.

FURTHER READING

• Curzio, J. Funding for evidence-based nursing practice in the UK. *Nursing Times Research* 1998; 3: 2, 100–107.

• Deighan, M., Boyd, K. Defining evidence-based health care: A health-care learning strategy? *Nursing Times Research* 1996; 1: 5, 332–339.

• Jenkinson, C. *Assessment and Evaluation in Health Care*. Buckingham: Open University Press, 1998.

• Muir, Gray, J.A. *Evidence-based Healthcare*. London: Churchill Livingstone, 1997.

• NHS Executive. *Promoting Clinical Effectiveness: A framework for action in and throughout the NHS*. London: Department of Health, 1996.

• Ovretveit, J. *Evaluating Health Interventions*. Buckingham: Open University Press, 1998.

• Salvage, J. Evidence-based practice: A mixture of motives. *Nursing Times* 1998; **94**: 23, 61–64.

• Schutz, A. The stranger: An essay in social psychology. In: Brodesen, A. (ed) *Studies in Social Theory (Collected Papers II)*. The Hague: Martinus Nijhoff, 1964.

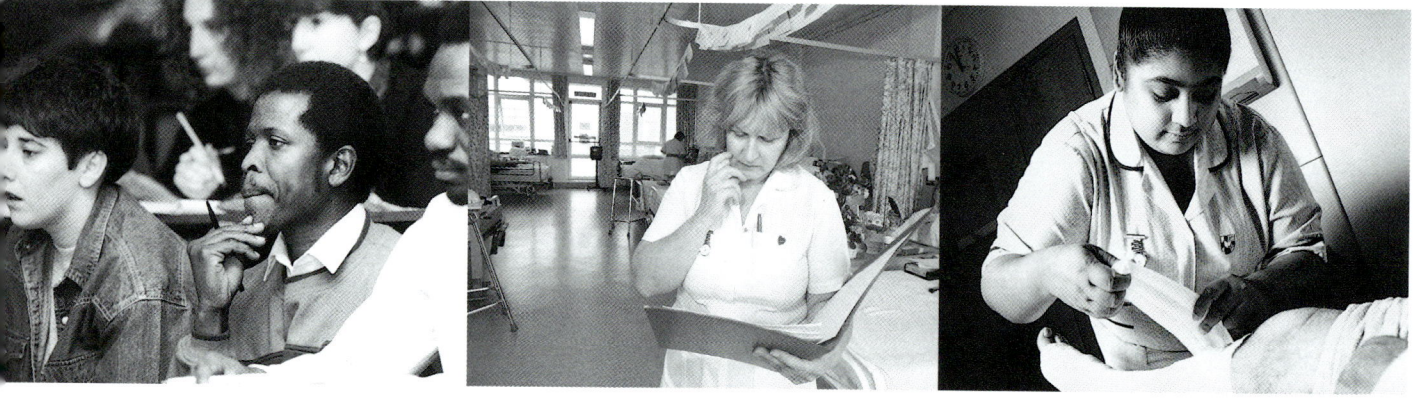

Notes

Rubbing shoulders with research

If you want to expand the research base of your nursing practice you need a strategy for reading and hearing about research. In this Part we explore ways in which you can increase your familiarity with research knowledge. You will:

- Read and assess a variety of media, from research journals to textbooks

- Look at the value of a journal club

- Watch a research-based videotape (if one is available to you) or attend a conference (if practical).

WORK PLANNER

Activities 3 and 5 ask you to look in detail at different sources of research-based knowledge: you are asked to locate and use material from journals and books.

We suggest that you find the sources before beginning this piece of work, in case of any delays in getting the material from your library.

You may find that this work is fairly time-consuming, or that you need to spread it over a larger period of time to get the maximum benefit from it.

Activity 6 asks you to watch a research-based videotape. Make inquiries early on to see if one is available.

You may want to refer to your Student Support Pack on using library resources.

USING OPPORTUNITIES

ACTIVITY 1
diary
Make some brief notes in your diary about all the current activities you consciously undertake to increase your stock of research-based knowledge. If you can't think of any, can you give reasons why not?

Many everyday nursing situations offer opportunities to help you develop practice which is more research-based. (*R1: Nursing: A Research-based Profession* and *R2(i): Sources of knowledge* summarised the principles of evidence-based practice).

Look at the following scenarios and decide whether or not you might be Nurse Keen.

Opportunity 1

Nurse: I've come to dress the wound on your foot, Mrs Clark. You know the routine by now, don't you?

Mrs Clark: Oh yes. Mind you, that other nurse who comes does it differently from you — uses different lotions as well, I think.

Nurse: Really? *(Thinks: Why does she always have to be different? It always causes trouble.)*

OR

Nurse Keen: That's interesting. Perhaps she heard of something new which works better. I'll check with her before I come back next week.

Opportunity 2

Nurse: I've come to help out because you're short-staffed on here. Where's Sister?

Ward clerk: You're a welcome sight. But we've introduced primary nursing here, so you'll need to see the ward co-ordinator — Sister is with her patients.

Nurse: OK *(Thinks: Not another new-fangled way of organising work — it never works when they're short-staffed.)*

OR

Nurse Keen: That's interesting. I haven't worked with a primary nursing system before. Have you got any research articles on it which I could read at lunchtime?

Opportunity 3

Nurse: Hello. You look very official clutching all those forms. What's up?

Student: We're doing a research project to investigate the patients' views on aromatherapy. Don't worry, it's all official and we've had the lecture from Sister about not getting under the nurses' feet.

Nurse: Thank goodness — for a terrible moment I thought you wanted me to dish the forms out.

OR

Nurse Keen: Now I come to think about it, Sister did tell us about it, but she didn't really tell us what it was for and what methods of data collection you are using. I can't stop now but I would love to hear about it — why don't you come to coffee and explain it all?

You can probably think of many other examples of commonplace nursing situations which you could use more creatively to 'rub shoulders with research'. The next Activity asks you to think about some of these.

83

ACTIVITY 2
diary
List any situations over the past week in your own nursing practice which offered you an opportunity to look into a piece of research. Were you able to use the research findings? If so, make a few notes on the outcomes of using them. Or note down why you couldn't use them.

Such spontaneous occasions cannot be the entire basis of your research-based knowledge. In order to underpin the standards you set for your practice, the knowledge you use has to be acquired more systematically.

As explained in *R2(i): Sources of knowledge*, much of our knowledge comes from two different types of source:

- Media — books, journals, videotapes, newsletters, the Internet.

- People — nurses, non-nursing colleagues, consultants, visiting lecturers, conferences, workshops.

Research knowledge is no exception, although some channels of communication or ways of *disseminating* (spreading) information are used by researchers more commonly than others. Next, we explore different sources of research-based knowledge that you might want to use.

MEDIA

We ask you now to think about how you might increase your contacts with research. If you have anxieties about your understanding of research, the best way to gain confidence is to increase your familiarity with it. By doing this, you may find that many of your questions will be answered without your having to ask them directly. Furthermore, you will feel more confident about seeking advice and help.

Don't be daunted by the following list of media. The idea is that you become comfortable with journals and the process of retrieving information. You don't need to get too bogged down in details at this stage.

The media used to disseminate research-based knowledge include:

- Research journals

- Research monographs

- Collections of research articles

- Research conference proceedings

- Research-based videotapes (where these are available)

- Research dissertations and theses

- Textbooks.

All of these, except the dissertations and theses, are published and available to the general public. Research dissertations and theses are unpublished, but they are available through the library service. You have to order them through the librarian and there may be particular constraints on the copyright; that is, you may not quote from them without special permission. The RCN library has a collection of nursing theses and monographs.

Many nurses are familiar with these sources, and if you are a conversion programme student you may have been using some of them already. However, it is useful to review them systematically so that you can organise your own reading routines — reading research can be very time-consuming, and it is not possible for anyone to read everything.

Activities 3–7 will help you to be selective in your reading. You will look at different media sources in turn.

Notes

RESEARCH JOURNALS

ACTIVITY 3
action
Find a recent issue of three different research journals; the three most commonly available are probably *Nursing Times Research*, the *Journal of Advanced Nursing* and *International Journal of Nursing Studies*. Look at them carefully and answer the following questions about each:
- What is the system of *refereeing* articles (selecting them for publication and checking their accuracy)?
- What kinds of articles are they asking contributors to submit?
- For each of the articles in that issue, make a note, using the *abstract* (that is, the summary at the beginning, rather than reading the whole article), of its likely relevance to your practice.
- Make notes of your impression of the whole issue of the journal; for example, its readability, relevance, presentation, inclusion of statistics
- Choose the article you think is most likely to be relevant, and read it. Note your impressions of the article which you read; for example, how well you could understand it, how relevant it was to practice, how long it took to read.

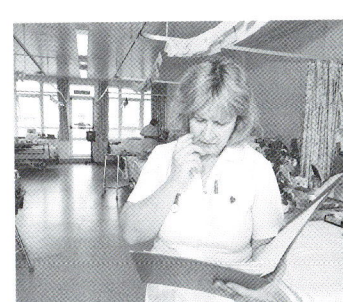

Reading a research journal can be fairly time-consuming if you are to grasp the important points and make a reasonable assessment of it. You will probably find it best to set aside at least half-an-hour for a first reading of an article, and then to read it two or three more times.

For an article that is important to an area of particular interest, you might want to go back to it several months later to check that you haven't forgotten some issues and to see if your initial assessment was correct. Usually your ideas change as you read and understand more about a topic or have new experiences, and this new perspective may change your assessment of an article.

Research Monographs and Collections of Research Articles

Activity 4 asks you to repeat the 'find and assess' process used above, this time with research monographs and collections of research articles — again, you may want to spread the work over a longer period of time than we suggested above.

Research monographs are usually accounts of a single piece of research. You may be familiar with the monographs in the RCN Research Series. *Collections of research articles* are usually focused on a particular theme; for example, the 'Developments in Nursing Research' volumes published by John Wiley & Sons Ltd include 'Psychiatric Nursing Research', 'Research in the Nursing Care of Elderly People', and 'Nursing Issues in Terminal Care' among their titles.

Notes

ACTIVITY 4
action
1. Find a research monograph which seems to be relevant to your area of practice. Skim through it and write notes in your diary on your initial reactions to it. Is it written in language that you can understand? Now read it carefully and make more notes of your opinions after more detailed consideration. Compare your first impressions with your thoughts after you have finished it.
2. Find a selection of research articles which seem relevant to your area of practice. Again, skim through them and make notes of your first impressions, then read the article which seems to be the most relevant, and the article which seems to be least relevant, to your practice. Compare your notes before and after your reading.

Research Conference Proceedings

These include all or most of the research papers read at a conference (an account of research which the researcher reads out at a conference or workshop is known as a *paper*). Such papers are harder to find in nursing than in other disciplines. It might, therefore, be easier to find the proceedings of a medical research conference.

ACTIVITY 5
action
If you can find the proceedings of a medical research conference, evaluate it in the same way as you did in the previous Activity for the research monographs and articles.

Research-based Videotapes

Videos are a fairly new source of research-based knowledge, and are not in widespread use as yet. However, North West Thames Regional Health Authority has published *Anything for Pain?*, a videotape presentation of research work on post-operative experience of pain. It was a deliberate attempt to improve the dissemination of research findings:

'The research-based video took under six months from planning to launch, which means that the research findings can become widely available in a relatively short period of time. It represents a new approach in the dissemination of nursing research and, hopefully, will help to bridge that much discussed gap between research and nursing practice'[1].

Research Dissertations and Theses

ACTIVITY 6
action
Try to find a videotape on nursing practice. Make notes in your diary on the research base of the information.
If you are able to watch the video with one or two colleagues, spend 10 minutes or so after watching it to discuss the approach taken to the subject and its usefulness in opening up research to you.

These are accounts of research work which are produced specifically by the researcher as part of the process of getting a degree. A dissertation is shorter than a thesis and is usually submitted as part of the work for a master's degree, which may also include taught courses and other types of assessment.

A thesis is a more substantial piece of work and usually represents the major work for a research degree, which may be awarded at two levels — master's level or doctoral. Because of the context in which a thesis is produced, it is not always very easy to read or understand — it was, after all, written to persuade the examiners, who are already experts in the subject, of how much the author knows, not to help people who know little about the subject to understand it. Nevertheless, you may need to consult a thesis or dissertation and it is useful to know how to get hold of one. As they must be ordered through a library, talk with your librarian about how to get information about them and how to order them.

Textbooks

Textbooks are perhaps the most difficult of all to read in terms of research, because they do not always make it clear which bits of information are research-based and which are not.

ACTIVITY 7
knowledge base
The box below contains an extract from a nursing textbook[2]. Read the extract and make a note of which information you think is based on research and which is not.

A change strategy

A full discussion of change theory and application is beyond the scope of this text and is covered elsewhere in detail (Wright, 1989). However, a number of key features can be identified here.

If, in accepting Ottoway's (1976) approach, then those who are working at nursing's grass roots — the ward staff, community nurses for example — must be the starting point for the process of change. In this instance, specific change agent roles (Ottoway, 1980) were created, persons charged with a remit to make changes, to concurrently affect both care and learning. The creation of a joint appointment ... was a calculated act to help tackle the thorny problem of the theory versus practice gap in nursing ... This is not a new idea; a report by Bell (1950) encapsulated the conflict for students when confronted with the approach —'You may have learned it like that in the classroom, but that's not how it's done in the wards'. Many well-researched detrimental effects, upon both students and teacher and ultimately upon the care the patient receives, have been documented as a result (Birch, 1974; Bendall, 1975; Kramer, 1974; Gott, 1984; Alexander, 1983).

FEEDBACK

This Activity is not an easy one to do, because the extract doesn't give us enough information. Although there is a sprinkling of references in the text we cannot always know whether they refer to research findings or to other types of knowledge. Sometimes the authors of texts are specific, and refer to 'Research by Bloggs et al. (1998) which shows ...' or 'Research findings (Bloggs 1998) suggest ...'. In our example above, we have the phrase 'many well-researched detrimental effects', followed by a number of references, so it is a reasonable assumption that these refer to research. When we turn to the list of references (reproduced below) to check we find this difficult to confirm, although it seems likely that most of them are published within the *RCN Research Monograph* series and can easily be checked; other books may need to be sent for and checked individually.

Birch, J. *To Nurse or Not to Nurse*. London: Royal College of Nursing, 1974.

Bendall, E. *So You Passed, Nurse*. London: Royal College of Nursing, 1975.

Kramer, M. *Reality Shock*. St Louis: Mosby, 1974.

Gott, M. *Learning Nursing*. London: Royal College of Nursing, 1984.

Alexander, M. F. *Learning to Nurse*. Edinburgh: Churchill Livingstone, 1983.

However, we are still left with Wright 1989, Ottoway 1976 and 1980, and Bell 1950. Here are the references in full:

Wright, S. G. *Changing Nursing Practice*. London: Edward Arnold, 1989.

Ottoway, R. N. A change strategy to implement new norms, new style and new environment in the work organisation. *Personnel Review* **5**: 1, Winter 1976.

Ottoway, R. N. *Defining the Change Agent*. Unpublished research paper, University of Manchester Institute of Technology, Department of Management Sciences, Manchester, 1980.

Bell, G. M. Report of the annual general meeting of the ward and departmental sisters' section of the Royal College of Nursing. *Nursing Times* 1950; **46**: 753–55.

ACTIVITY 8
action
Underline those references in the above list which you are now confident refer to research.

The above example shows why identifying research-based information in general textbooks may not be an easy task. The task is made more difficult by the conventions which apply to different disciplines. Look at the passage below from a nursing textbook on physiology[3].

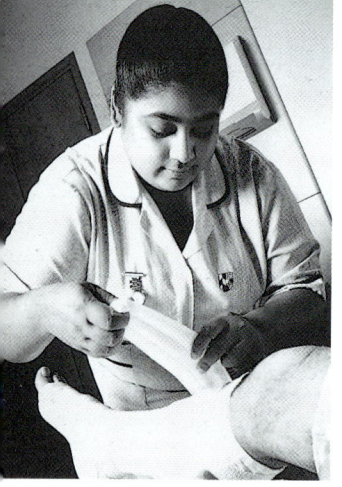

Body water

Water is by far the largest single component of the body because it makes up 45 – 75% of the total body weight ... Infants have the highest percentage of water, up to 75% of body weight. This percentage decreases with age. Since adipose tissue (fat) contains almost no water, fat people have a smaller proportion of water than do lean people. In a normal adult male, water accounts for about 60% of body weight. Because females, on average, have more subcutaneous fat than males, their total body water is lower, accounting for about 55% of body weight.

You will have noticed that there are no references to sources in the passage at all, yet we can confidently assert that all the information is research-based. This is because within the natural sciences there is considerable agreement about a great deal of the research-based knowledge which forms the 'core' knowledge of the discipline, and it is acceptable not to reference the original source. References will still be used where there are areas of doubt or disagreement, or where the research work is relatively recent. In a discipline such as sociology or psychology, there is far less agreement about a central body of knowledge, so considerably more referencing is conventionally used, even of research texts which are many years old.

Because the knowledge isn't referenced it is most important that you use an up-to-date physiology book. Older books in subjects such as psychology and sociology can still be useful because they define their references, although you may have to add to your knowledge with some more up-to-date reading.

Written sources have the great value of usually being available at a time and place which suits you. Obviously there are exceptions — you may have to wait for books to arrive from the inter-library loan service, and most theses can be used only in a library. However, generally speaking, written sources are accessible — an advantage which students of the conversion programme will be familiar with. But they have one great disadvantage — you cannot ask them questions if you don't understand something. An actual researcher 'in the flesh', though, can be interrogated, points can be clarified and additional information can be sought. Moreover, if the point is not clear, the researcher can be asked to explore with you the relevance of his/her work to your practical concerns.

Journal Clubs

Because keeping up to date with a range of research journals takes far more time than most nurse practitioners have available, journal clubs have been formed. These are groups of nurses who meet regularly and share information about what they have read; usually each member agrees to read one journal, knowing that her colleagues will tell her what she has missed in the others. Figure 1 describes how one journal club is organised.

Fig 1. An example of information provided to practitioners about a local journal club. (Reproduced with the kind permission of Mrs J. Blake, nurse teacher — Care of the Elderly, Powys, Health Authority)

Running a Journal Club

The purpose of a Journal Club is to provide an opportunity for nurses who are interested in keeping up to date with the latest developments and research in nursing to meet together on an informal basis.

The Club meets on the first Tuesday of every month, after an early shift, over coffee and biscuits. It is held in the Resources Room of the Teaching Unit, which offers comfortable chairs and a quiet environment away from the ward.

Each Club member, if he/she so wishes, takes it in turn to be responsible for reading a nursing journal or a healthcare journal for a month. All the journals are available in the hospital library. Those members then bring along to the meeting a summary of one or two articles which they have found to be of particular interest or use, and use them for group discussion.

Club members usually rotate the responsibility for reading different journals each month. There is no pressure, though, on all members to take responsibility for reading a journal. Nurses may attend merely to listen to the summaries and join in the group discussions. The best individual benefit is derived from the Club, however, when one takes an active role.

This sharing and discussing of articles enables all club members to keep in touch with the large selection of journals available to nurses today.

ACTIVITY 9
action
If you already attend a journal club, list the reasons why you find it useful. If you do not find it particularly helpful make a note of the reasons why — perhaps you do not attend regularly enough.
Are there any recommendations you could make to the club?
If you do not attend a journal club, find out the details of a local club and arrange to attend meetings. Or you might consider organising a group of colleagues — perhaps the staff in your ward — into a journal club.
Your tutor may be able to help you start up a journal club.

Notes

MEETING RESEARCHERS

The best places to meet researchers working in your area of interest are at:

- Conferences and workshops

- Courses

- Research interest groups within and outside your workplace.

Conferences and workshops are widely advertised and can be very useful. As well as being able to discuss research findings with researchers at these, you will also meet practitioners with interests similar to yours and a network of contacts can be built up. Courses — especially short courses of one and two days — operate similarly.

Research interest groups vary widely between areas. Usually they invite researchers to talk about their work — either completed research or work in progress — and provide plenty of opportunity for discussion and for clarifying straightforward points. Activity 10 asks you to think about one particular way of increasing your contact with the people who do research in an area of practice which interests you.

As you work through the programme, look out for other opportunities to increase your contact with researchers through conferences, workshops or research groups.

ACTIVITY 10
action
Look through back copies of *Nursing Times* until you find an advertisement for a research conference/workshop which you would have liked to attend. Make a note of why you think it would have been relevant to your practice and what you could have contributed to your team if you had gone.

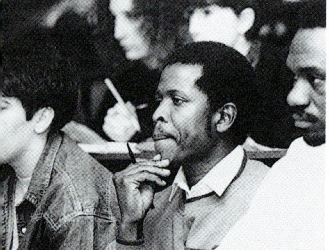

FOCUS

Look back over the variety of activities you have done here. Now draw up an action plan for yourself. The aim of your plan is to ensure that you are regularly reading and hearing about research. Starting points for your action plan could be:

- Allocating reading time during your week

- Joining or setting up a journal club

- Planning ahead to attend workshops/seminars.

Talk to your tutor and your colleagues about your plan — they may be able to help you on practical points or tell you about local opportunities.

REFERENCES

1 Seers, K. Perceptions of pain. *Nursing Times* 1987; **83**: 48, 37–39.
2 Wright, S. *Building and Using a Model of Nursing.* (2nd edn.) London: Edward Arnold, 1990.
3 Tortora, C.J., Grabowski, S. Reynolds. *Principles of Anatomy and Physiology.* (8th edn.) New York: HarperCollins, 1996.

FURTHER READING

- Couchman, W., Dawson, J. *New rituals for old: Nursing through the looking glass.* Oxford: Butterworth-Heinemann, 1994.
- Owen, D., Davis, M. Help with your project. (2nd edn.) London: Edward Arnold, 1997.
- Scharr Website: http://www.shef.ac.uk/~scharr/ir/netting.html
- Smaje, C. *Health, Race and Ethnicity: Making sense of the evidence.* London: King's Fund Institute 1995.
- Smith, P. (ed). *Research Mindedness for Practice: An interactive approach for nursing and healthcare.* Edinburgh: Churchill Livingston, 1997.

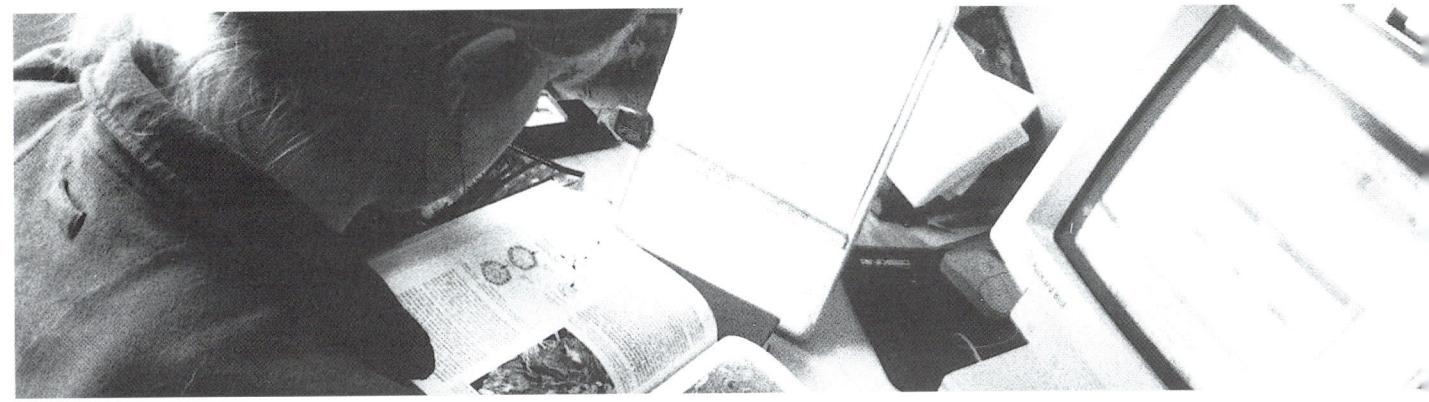

Reading research reports

R2(i): Sources of knowledge and *R2(ii): Rubbing shoulders with research* looked at why and how you might increase or enhance your knowledge base by seeking out research-based knowledge. In this Part we take you through a step-by-step approach to reading a research report.

You will look at:

- The way a research report is set out
- How to identify the purpose and strategy of the report
- Different sorts of data used in research reports
- How data are analysed
- Ethical problems facing the reader
- How relevant the research report is to you and to your patients
- The importance of research findings for evidence-based practice.

WORK PLANNER

For this Part we would like you to use two reasonably short reports. Make sure they are articles, rather than research monographs, preferably from two different journals.

We suggest you use your usual system of making notes and a system of filing them so that you can find the information easily when you need it.

The following are suggestions for filing which you might want to adopt.

- Keep your notes about an article on the back of the record card (easiest if you use the biggest size of card) on which the details of the article are written

- If the notes are too long to fit on the card, you can write on A4 sheets and staple them onto the back of the card

- If the article is in a book, file the notes in the filing cabinet as if they were the article. For example, notes on an article by Bloggins would be filed under B and the record card on Bloggins' article would have a note to that effect.

MAKING A START

This Part of *R2: Focusing on Research Knowledge* takes you through the stages of reading a research report. The process we will describe is simple and straightforward and should provide a useful guide. But you don't have to follow the steps or stages in this order or indeed at all. If you already have a tried and tested way of reading and understanding research reports, we don't recommend that you change your style now. But if you aren't too familiar with research reports then this might be a good foundation, to which we will be adding in future Parts.

It is usually best to start by reading the article all the way through without making any notes at all, or perhaps just highlighting a couple of key words as you go through. Sometimes you can cut short the whole process at this stage by deciding that the article is no use, and throwing it in the bin. This doesn't happen very often but occasionally you request an article which looks as though it is going to be about nursing — 'Caring for the newborn in difficult circumstances', for example — and it turns out to be about the lambing season in Outer Mongolia. More likely, you discover that it isn't a research report at all but a summary of knowledge taken from other places. This may be very useful but, as we saw in R2(ii), it needs to be read slightly differently from a research report. But more usually you realise that the article is a research report, and that it says important things, and so you need to read it more carefully.

READING REPORTS: A STRATEGY

The following is a strategy for reading which should enable you to read objectively and critically, and to judge the value to you of any research report.

Research Conventions

The reporting of research is done in a highly conventional way. The conventions of report-writing may have a tendency to 'tidy up' the picture, so that the reader doesn't always get a feel for the complexities and difficulties of carrying out research. Nevertheless, most articles will follow a format similar to that below[1].

- **Introduction** — This gives the background to the study and tells you why the particular piece of research was undertaken. A brief summary of previous and related work will also be given — either in the introduction or possibly under a separate heading: Literature Review

- **Method** — a description of how the study was carried out

- **Results** — the results of the study

- **Discussion** — The results are discussed by the author of the report in the light of previous work and other relevant issues

- **Conclusion** — The author summarises the study, drawing the threads together and perhaps indicating the uses or implications of the study

- **References** — All the studies mentioned in the text are listed in detail. You should be able to find these relatively easily if the references have been presented correctly

- **Appendices** — contain material of interest, relevant to the study itself, but not included in the body of the report (for example, the questionnaire or interview schedule used for doing the research).

To read an article critically and analytically you may find it helpful to ask a series of questions which cut across the sections which the author is using. By doing that you can avoid the temptation to see the work in the same way as the author. These questions are:

- What is it for?

- What was the overall strategy?

- What sorts of data were produced?

- How were the data analysed?

- Does this report present me with any ethical problems?

- What is the relevance of this work for me (and my patients)?

What is it for?

First ask yourself some questions about the whole study. What was the purpose behind the study? What were the aims of the researcher? *What is it for?* There may be more than one aspect to this. First, there are the reasons why this topic was chosen. For example, the researcher may claim it is a different way of looking at an old problem; or, conversely, the topic may have been chosen because no one has looked at it before.

The second aspect is why the researcher is doing the research. Is this the researcher's job? Does the researcher have an overwhelming interest in the topic? Is it part of work for a higher degree?

A third aspect is to consider who paid for the research to be done. It may have been the health service, a government body, a company involved in the healthcare market, a charity, or indeed the researcher may have funded much of it through providing his/her own time.

None of the answers to these questions will necessarily make the conclusions of the study less valid, but they do indicate the constraints within which the research was carried out. We will be investigating the effects of such constraints in a later Part in the Research Module.

> **ACTIVITY 1**
> **knowledge base**
> Read both of your chosen reports. Make notes for both of them in answer to the questions:
> - What is the purpose of the research?
> - What is the purpose of the researcher?
> - Who funded the research?

You may have found very little information about these aspects in your reports. If you have looked carefully then don't worry — not all research reports provide the same information, although it might be more helpful to us as consumers if they did.

What was the overall strategy?

How did the researcher go about her business? What was her overall strategy? Did she, for example, decide to observe things without getting involved? Did she decide to get involved and hope that would give her ideas about what was going on? Did she ask other people what was going on? Did she make any systematic changes to what was going on before she started her work?

Let's look at an example, from some work by Metcalf[2]:

> The present study involves the introduction of a system of Patient Allocation (in this case Team Nursing) into a ward of a Maternity Hospital.
>
> As in the before-mentioned studies, the following reputed advantages of a change to a system of Patient Allocation will be investigated:
>
> 1. That the nurses obtain greater job satisfaction
>
> 2. That the patients will be more satisfied with the care that they receive.
>
> In this study, however, the approach is different in that it is not only designed to test hypotheses, but is also explanation-generating in an attempt to discover and understand the process of introducing change. What is important to understand is how a system of Patient Allocation is interpreted by the nurses and by the patients — what it is in practice and what it means for both.
>
> The theoretical framework being adopted here is that when undertaking an evaluation of a planned organisational change which affects both nursing staff and patient roles in an organisation such as a hospital, it is important to examine the orientations of both nursing staff and patients before, during and after the change. Important among these orientations are the expectations that staff have of their work and the expectations that patients have of their stay.

Notes

The explanation above of the research study uses some fairly complicated language, but if we read it carefully, we can see that it provides answers to our first two questions above.

ACTIVITY 2

knowledge base

Underline those passages in the previous extract which indicate:
- Why Metcalf wants to do this study. What is different about it compared with others?
- What her overall approach is. Is she comparing X with Y? In whose thoughts is she interested? What sort of statement does she want to be able to make at the end?

FEEDBACK

We would have underlined '*the approach is different ... is also explanation-generating*'; this indicates that Metcalf obviously thinks she can add an extra dimension to previous work .

We would also have underlined '*... attempt to discover and understand the processes of introducing change ... to understand how ... is interpreted by the nurses and patients ... to examine the orientations before, during and after the change ...*' because they offer an understanding of what the overall approach will be — to explore what nurses' and patients' understanding is of what is going on, not to test some ideas of the researcher. The exact words which you underline are not important, but it is important to 'cut through' some of the wordiness which research reports often include, in order to get to the heart of the approach. You may not have understood some of the words used in the quoted extract (for example, 'hypotheses'), but this won't necessarily have prevented you from understanding the approach.

ACTIVITY 3

knowledge base

Look through your two research reports again, and for both make a note, either by underlining (if it is your copy), or by jotting down those words which convey an understanding of the whole approach used by the researcher. Then write a note summarising the approach of each article.

Try not to get too involved with the intricacies of the research design, or with the research terminology. Avoid writing things such as *It is a questionnaire design*, or *It is an observational study*, but try to use simple words, for example, *The researcher is asking them what they do*, or, *The researcher is observing what they do*.

What sorts of data were produced?

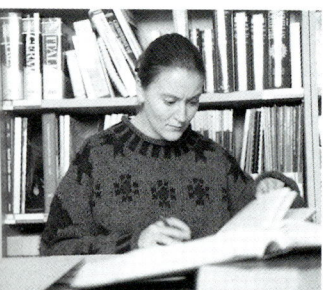

What were the data which the researcher used for the analysis? 'Data' is another term for information or evidence, and a lot of research involves generating new data.

EXAMPLES

One researcher tape-recorded visits by health visitors to mothers with very young babies. The data were the tape recordings, which would not have existed if she had not made them.

Other research might ask clients about the services they receive; the answers would be the new data.

Or a researcher might measure the growth of bacteria in a wound. The figures generated would be the new data.

In Metcalf's study she had a staff satisfaction survey — so she generated statements about the staff's satisfaction. She also used a patient satisfaction survey — which again generated statements. And she included an observational study which generated information about a number of nursing activities such as the time spent on interacting with patients (in the form of measurements), and descriptions of what they did (such as the observation that they used work-books).

New data produced by researchers are known as *primary data*. Primary data are the data which researchers interpret to produce their conclusions.

These conclusions may themselves be used by other researchers, and be reinterpreted to form different conclusions. Used in this way, the conclusions are known as *secondary data*. Secondary data can also include material such as patient records, which consist of a number of items of primary data (name, age, condition and so on) interpreted in a specific way (the record) to suit the needs of healthcare professionals.

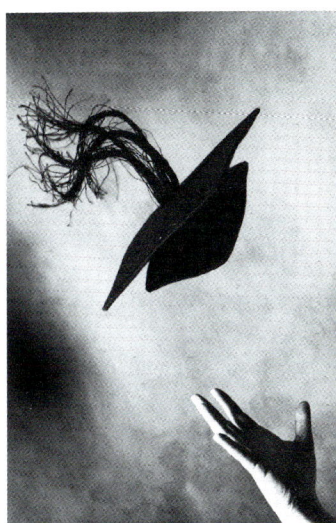

ACTIVITY 4
knowledge base
For both of your reports make notes on:
• The type of data collected, for example, written answers to questions, tape-recorded natural conversation, recorded numbers of something
• Whether the data are primary or secondary.

Any data, whether primary or secondary, are satisfactory provided they fit the purpose for which they are being used[3]. But sometimes data are used inappropriately, or in place of another type of data which would have been more useful. For example, suppose that you wanted to know if your patients enjoy their meals. You could:

• Ask them yourself

• Give them a written questionnaire to complete

• Ask their relatives

• Observe them as they are eating

• Check how much food remained on their plates.

ACTIVITY 5
diary
What problems could you foresee with using the types of data listed above in gaining accurate information about whether your patients enjoyed their meals?

FEEDBACK

Your answer will depend on your patients and your situation. Some of the difficulties would be: Are your patients able to complete a questionnaire? Are their relatives reliable witnesses? Are you actually there when they eat their meals, or are you long gone to the next client? You might also have thought about why asking your patients directly might not produce an accurate picture of their opinions of their meals.

ACTIVITY 6
knowledge base
Look again at the data in your reports. Do you think the data were the most useful in the circumstances? Would other data have given a more accurate picture? If you think other types of data would have been more useful, consider whether there were reasons why it might not have been possible to collect it.

FEEDBACK

Sometimes a researcher knows other data would give a more accurate picture but it does not seem feasible for ethical or practical reasons to collect them. For example, if we want to know about people's sexual habits, a video camera in every bedroom (and bathroom and garden shed) would produce the most accurate data, but usually researchers confine themselves to asking questions instead.

Before we leave the subject of data, think about whether the researcher used all the data collected. If not, why not?

ACTIVITY 7
knowledge base
Did the researcher use all the data collected for the analysis? If she didn't, does she say why? Check your reports again and make notes.

How were the data analysed?

In order to reach some conclusions, the researcher will have to do things with the data. As a minimum, she might add them together and come up with a result, for example, '64 patients said they hated injections and four said they enjoyed them.' Or she might do some simple statistics, for example: 'Of a group of 30, 90% of the patients said they wanted to go home. Of the remaining 10%, 6% didn't know and 4% didn't have a home.'

Notes

Try not to worry when reading statistics. You may sometimes see different letters and numbers, the most common being 'N' values and 'P' values. These are simply a way of proving significance. N means the number involved, and P means the probability of its occurring again — its significance. The lower the P value, the more significant. So if P is 00.05 or less, it is significant. For example: P=00.01 is highly significant. P=00.15 is not significant.

It is useful to have a simple statistics book to hand to help you understand if the correct test has been used for the sample size, and to understand significance.

ACTIVITY 8
knowledge base
For both reports, describe in your own words (that is, don't worry about getting the research jargon right) what the researcher 'did' to the data.

The results of the analysis will lead (it is hoped) to some conclusions. In the next Activity, we want you to think about how the conclusions relate to the analysis; for example, the conclusion might be that the analysis didn't prove anything, or that the question was asked wrongly in the first place.

ACTIVITY 9
knowledge base
For your reports, describe in your own words how the conclusions reached by the author relate to what he/she found out in the analysis.

Does this report present me with any ethical problems?

The issue of ethics can be a major problem for researchers. Research is an inherently nosy activity and it is not always clear where to draw the line, especially as patients are usually only too ready to talk. You may have had some direct experience of this problem during your work in earlier Parts when you were asked to carry out interviews with various individuals. But we are talking here about reading research, not doing research. What are your particular problems as a reader?

ACTIVITY 10
discussion
If you read an account which you believe describes unethical behaviour, what action will you take? Tick one or more of the list below.
• Write to the researcher
• Write to the journal or publisher
• Throw it in the bin
• Report it to the UKCC
• Use the results.
Discuss your actions with one or two colleagues or others in your study group. What are their views about how to deal with any unethical behaviour described in a published account? Explore each others' reasons.

FEEDBACK

While there are many texts which discuss the ethical dilemmas of the researcher, there seems to be little advice on the ethical dilemma of the reader.

You may have felt that you should write to the researcher first, because the account of the research may have misrepresented — perhaps for reasons of space in a journal — what was actually done. If it was in a journal you might also write to the editor — most journals have codes of practice about excluding unethical research. But there remains a real problem, which is exemplified by accounts of the research done on concentration camp inmates during the Second World War. While the research was clearly unethical — many of the research subjects died horribly in the course of the research — much of the analysis and data were recovered after the war and used as the basis for effective patient care in the years that followed.

ACTIVITY 11
discussion
There is a body of work on the effects of low temperature on the body which was carried out — often with fatal results — on prisoners in concentration camps. Would you knowingly use the results of that research to treat patients with hypothermia in your care?

You may want to discuss this issue, or any other ethical issues which arise from the research reports you read, with other students or colleagues. We will be considering some more general issues relating to ethics and nursing in a later Section.

Is the work relevant to me (and my patients)?

You are reading research with the aim of improving your practice. Does the researcher make any specific references to how the work can be used in practice? If so, how do they relate to your practice? Care might be needed here to avoid rejecting research out of hand. Metcalf's study, for example, was entitled: 'Patient Allocation in a Maternity Ward: A report of some of the findings', so if you are not working in a maternity ward you might think it does not apply to you. But if you read through the example again you will find that she is dealing with a more general issue: an attempt to discover *and understand the process of introducing change*. And of course this applies to all of us.

> **ACTIVITY 12**
> **knowledge base**
> For your research reports, make a note of:
> - Whether they contain any specific references to the implications for practice
> - The relationship with your own practice situation
> - What connections (if any) you can make to your own practice if there are no references at all to practice connections.

As you read through your research reports it will be obvious that, as well as having similarities, there are differences between them. Some of these differences relate to presentation, but there are also important differences in the way the research was done. We will be looking at the reasons for these differences in later Parts. Meanwhile, try to read as widely as you can, making detailed notes on your reading using the framework which we have explored here. You will eventually find that you have a bank of your own summaries of research which illustrate the range of research strategies. Don't reject any that are unfamiliar or difficult; just make a note of what seemed strange and why you found it difficult.

EVIDENCE-BASED PRACTICE AND RESEARCH

R1: Nursing: A Research-based Profession and *R2(i): Sources of knowledge* summarised the nature of evidence-based practice and its role in modern nursing practice. The use of research findings is one of the major ways research is translated into practice in evidence-based nursing.

FOCUS

Write a brief summary (not more then 200 words) of the reports which you have been using. Assume that you were trying to convey to someone who hadn't read them the *essence* of what they were about.

Give a copy of *one* of the articles, and your summary of it, to a friend or mentor. Ask that person to discuss with you how well your summary conveys the essential elements of the article.

REFERENCES

1   Ogier, M. *Reading Research*. London: Scutari, 1989.
2   Metcalf, C. A. Patient allocation in a maternity ward: A report of some of the findings. In: Redfern, S., Sisson, A. R., Walker J. E., Walsh P. A. (eds). *Issues in Nursing Research. Papers from the 22nd Annual Conference of the Royal College of Nursing Research Society*. London: Macmillan Press, 1982, pp 246–272.
3   While, A. Records as a data source. *Journal of Advanced Nursing* 1987; **12**: 157–163.

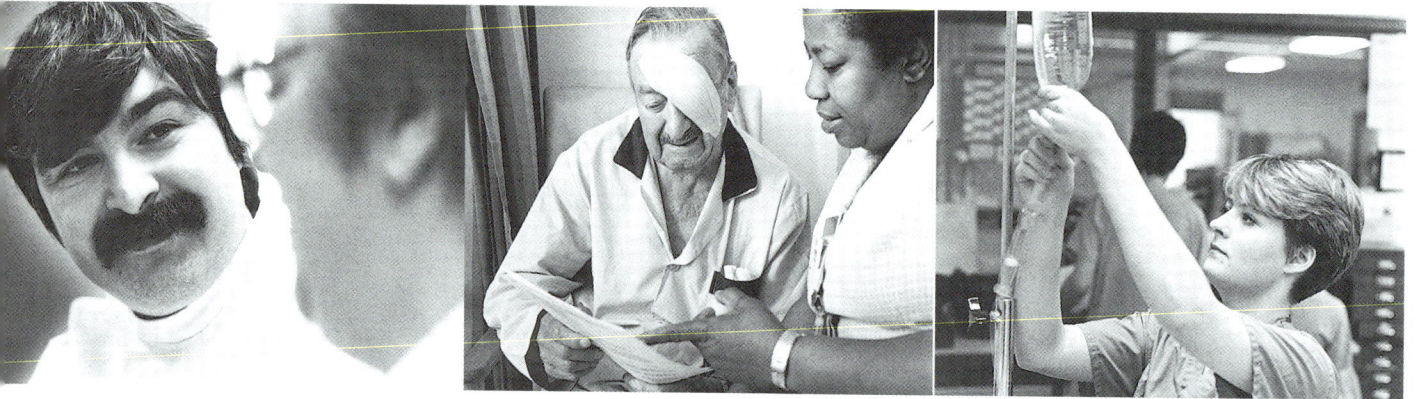

What is a registered nurse?

This Part looks at what it takes to make a 'registered nurse' and why we have a system of legal registration for nurses. It includes what the nursing role covers and how the profession maintains 'quality control' among its members.

In particular you will consider:

- The qualities and skills a nurse should have

- What other people think about nursing and how much weight their views should carry

- The purpose of registration

- Assessment for nurses

- The competences required for a second-level and a first-level nurse

- The code of professional conduct.

WORK PLANNER

You will need a copy of the UKCC *Code of Professional Conduct for the Nurse, Midwife and Health Visitor*, 3rd edition (1992), published by the UKCC. It is available free of charge from them.

WHAT IS A NURSE?

We start this debate by trying to define exactly what a nurse is, might or should be.

ACTIVITY 1
diary
In your diary, describe in a few sentences, or lists of words, what you think a nurse ought to be.

FEEDBACK

You could have used a number of criteria for your description. Did you set down a number of *qualities*, such as being kind, sympathetic, objective or organised? Did you go for *skills*, such as being able to cope well with emergencies or being able to handle sick people appropriately? Or did you describe *areas of knowledge*, such as that required to advise on general health promotion, or the prevention of the complications of immobility? Maybe you used all three criteria, to produce a fairly complex definition.

Nursing is an ancient occupation and there has been a long-term debate about what a nurse should be. Consider this 17th-century 'nurse specification', by Thomas Fuller[1]:

Of a nurse:

Though it is possible to meet with a Nurse every way so qualify'd for the Business as to have no Faults or Failings, yet the more she cometh up to the following Particulars the more she is to be liked. It is therefore desirable that she be,

1. Of a middle Age, fit and able to go through with the necessary Fatigue of her Undertaking.

2. Healthy, especially free from Vapours and Cough.

3. A good Watcher, that can hold fitting up the whole Course of the Sickness.

4. Quick in Hearing and always ready at the first Call.

5. Quiet and Still, so as to talk low, and but little, and tread softly.

6. Of good Sight to observe the Pocks, their Colour, Manner, and Growth, and all Alterations that may happen.

7. Handy to do Every Thing the best way, without Blundering and Noise.

8. Nimble and Quick a going, coming and doing Every Thing.

9. Cleanly, to make all she dresseth acceptable.

10. Well-tempered, to humour, and please the Sick as much as she can.

11. Chearful and Pleasant; to make the best of Every Thing, without being at any time Cross, Melancholy, or Timorous.

12. Constantly careful and diligent by Night and Day.

13. Sober and Temperate; not given to Gluttony, Drinking, or Smoaking.

14. Observant to follow the Physician's Orders duly; and not to be so conceited of her own Skill, as to give her own medicines privately.

15. To have no Children, or others to come much after her.

ACTIVITY 2
diary
In your diary, note down those qualities and skills from Thomas Fuller's list that you think you have.

We return to Thomas Fuller's list later on, but for the moment we are going to consider the ideas behind modern nursing and the legal registration that now prohibits anyone not registered from claiming to be a nurse.

IDEOLOGIES OF NURSING

An *ideology* is a set of ideas that reflect the beliefs and interests of a group with a common purpose. However, there are different views, and therefore different ideologies, of nursing, depending on the group looking at it.

ACTIVITY 3
diary
List different groups of people who might have a view on what nursing is. Make a few notes about what their views might be.

FEEDBACK

Doctors are one group who have a view on nursing. Thomas Fuller was a physician, and was putting forward a medical *ideology* of nursing, particularly noticeable in 'not be so conceited of her own Skill, as to give her own medicines privately'!

The public also has a view. What do they expect of nurses?

One survey, made during the development phase of this programme, asked a small sample of people from different age groups: 'What are nurses there for?' The response indicated that among the sample interviewed there was a strong belief that 'nurses do things for sick people under the instructions of the doctor'. These people were expressing an ideology which sees nursing as being under the direction of the medical profession, concerned solely with the sick, and made up entirely of practical skills.

Increasingly, however, people are beginning to change their views about what nurses do. Patients now see nurses as taking more responsibility for the care provided. Ask yourself what you, as a healthcare professional, look like from an outsider's point of view — that is, from the perspective of a patient or client.

The idea of nurses having their own body of knowledge, and a role which encompasses not only caring for the sick but also advising and encouraging people to do things for themselves, is more and more what the public believes a nurse should be.

ACTIVITY 4
diary
Who do you think should decide what role nurses play in society? Should the opinions of the public be given as much, or more, weight than the opinions of nurses in deciding what the profession should be and do?

One great problem about changes in nurse education, such as Project 2000, which was designed to prepare nurses more appropriately for their role, is that the changes may have been made by the profession without really knowing what the public wants from it. The decision as to what the nurse's role should be has been taken by nurses using a professional nursing ideology which may differ from the ideology of the people they care for.

A further problem lies in the fact that there are many different opinions within the nursing profession itself. The UKCC consulted widely before putting forward the final Project 2000 proposals[2], based on a professional nursing ideology, yet there are still many different opinions within the profession over the way Project 2000 has been implemented. We therefore have different ideologies of nursing, not only from different groups outside the nursing profession, such as doctors and possibly among the general public, but also within the profession itself. This diversity can be of great benefit, because it makes us question what, as a profession, we 'are'. It also means that in the process of questioning we must continually justify our existence as a profession.

ACTIVITY 5
diary
How effective do you think Project 2000 is in preparing people to become level-1 nurses? In what ways could it be improved?

REGISTRATION

The fact that nursing is recognisable as a profession, protected by Act of Parliament, is the result of the political activity of a group of militant nurses for a period of over 30 years before registration was finally achieved in 1919[3]. They united in a common aim, and their victory was described in the editorial of the *British Journal of Nursing* of 5th July 1919. In recent years the government has realised that more recognition needs to be given to the professional status of nursing. In September 1998, for example, it agreed a pay boost for nurses, midwives and health visitors.

The journal's editor, Mrs Bedford Fenwick, was one of the most militant and vocal nurses of the time, and she described the achievement of registration as:

'placing in the forefront registration of nurses, for the standardisation and improvement of nursing education, for the protection of the sick, and for the improvement of economic status of trained nurses'[4].

The legal basis for nurse registration today is laid down in the Nurses, Midwives and Health Visitors Act 1979[5]. The Act legislated for the establishment of new *statutory bodies* (groups whose existence is prescribed by law) for nursing: the *United Kingdom Central Council for Nursing, Midwifery and Health Visiting* (UKCC) and the four *National Boards for England, Scotland, Wales and Northern Ireland.*

The Act gave the UKCC the duty of establishing and improving standards of training and professional conduct for nurses, midwives and health visitors, and gave the boards the functions of providing, and being responsible for, the standards of courses of training leading to registration and for further training of those already registered.

The European Community

The task facing the UKCC in reforming nurse education in this country was complicated by Britain's membership of the European Community (now known as the European Union). Nurses training in member countries must meet a number of common training experiences. These are laid down in a European Community Council Directive[6] and cover not only the subjects and experiences essential to general nurse training programmes, but also the length of time of courses and the number of hours that they must include.

ACTIVITY 6
discussion
What difference do you think registration makes? What do you think the advantages are for yourself as a registered nurse or for any other groups or individuals? Make notes in your diary in answer to these questions and discuss your thoughts with friends and colleagues.

ASSESSMENT

How do we know when someone is competent to be registered as a nurse, and how do we ensure that that person's level of competence continues after registration? We need ways of *assessing* nursing ability that are relevant and 'real', and then *ensuring* that registered nurses maintain their levels of competence.

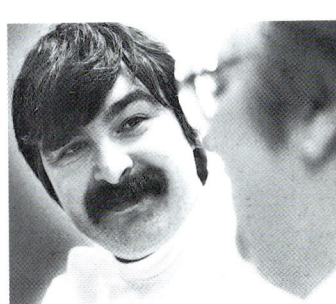

Assessment should not be a hurdle, a once-and-for-all experience which deters us from ever thinking about the course content and experience again. Assessment should be a useful tool that helps those being assessed to think, to learn and then to think again. In other words, it should be used to help us to become *reflective practitioners*, people going about the practice of nursing in an intelligent and thoughtful way. That is what we hope we have achieved with the assessment procedure for this course, in keeping with the idea that the nurse of the future will be a *knowledgeable doer*.

Levels of Competence

To achieve registration, and become one of the new 'knowledgeable doers', a nurse must meet a number of specific nursing competences. As a registered second-level nurse you are already required to meet one set of competences. They are set out in Rule 18(2) of the Nurses, Midwives and Health Visitors Rules Approval Order 1983[7].

Those relating to enrolled nurses are described as follows:

acquire the competences required to:

(a) assist in carrying out comprehensive observation of the patient and help in assessing her care requirements

(b) develop skills to enable her to assist in the implementation of nursing care under the direction of a person registered in parts 1, 3, 5 or 8 of the register

(c) accept delegated nursing tasks

(d) assist in reviewing the effectiveness of the care provided

(e) work in a team with other nurses, and with medical and paramedical staff and social workers.

Those registered in Parts 1, 3, 5 or 8 of the Register are level-1 nurses.

Notes

FEEDBACK

To be registered as a level-1 nurse you will need to:

acquire the competences required to:

(a) advise on the promotion of health and the prevention of illness

(b) recognise situations that may be detrimental to the health and well-being of the individual

(c) carry out those activities involved when conducting the comprehensive assessment of a person's nursing requirements

(d) recognise the significance of the observations made and use them to develop an initial nursing assessment

(e) devise a plan of nursing care based on the assessment with the co-operation of the patient, to the extent that this is possible, taking into account the medical prescription

(f) implement the planned programme of nursing care and, where appropriate, teach and co-ordinate other members of the caring team who may be responsible for implementing specific aspects of the nursing care

(g) review the effectiveness of the nursing care provided and, where appropriate, initiate any action that may be required

(h) work in a team with other nurses, and with medical and paramedical staff and social workers

(i) undertake the management of the care of a group of patients over a period of time and organise the appropriate support services.

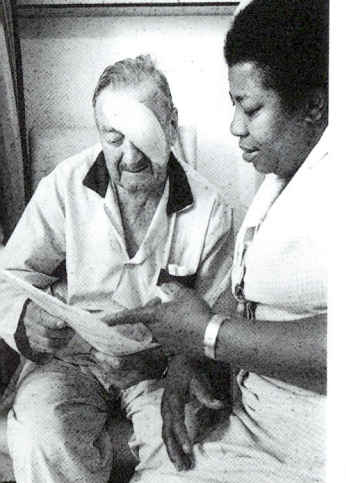

The competences of a level-1 nurse are examined in detail in *P4(ii): The competences in context*. What they could mean in your own field of nursing practice is also considered. We are now going to explore how these standards are maintained, by considering how a nurse is required to continue to meet competences in his or her work in the many years of practice that may follow registration at whatever level.

CODE OF PROFESSIONAL CONDUCT

The UKCC publishes a *Code of Professional Conduct for the Nurse, Midwife and Health Visitor*[8]. Serious failure to meet the standards of conduct listed in this document can result in the removal of a nurse's name from the register, thereby prohibiting him or her from practice.

There are quite a number of similarities between the 17th century ideology and the ideologies of today at which we have looked. This seems to indicate that, although ideologies may differ, there are some basic, and apparently enduring, areas of agreement about what a nurse should be and how a nurse should behave.

CASE STUDY

Tommy is elderly, has been an insulin-dependent diabetic for some years, and has peripheral neuropathy and poor eyesight. He also has chronic bronchitis, and from time to time acute exacerbations of this cause varying degrees of ketoacidosis if not very promptly treated. One night, Tommy's wife, Betty, woke up to hear him coughing and vomiting. When she tried to help him it became obvious that he was confused. Betty immediately called her son. She also called the doctor, who decided that Tommy had an acute chest infection, that his diabetic state needed careful monitoring and that he therefore required hospital care.

By this time, Tommy's son and daughter-in-law, Jim and Jenny, had arrived and they accompanied him to hospital. It was a bitterly cold night and Jim slipped on a large patch of ice outside the accident and emergency department. He pointed this out to the porter who came out to meet them with a wheelchair for Tommy, and the porter said: 'It's all right, mate, I know.'

Inside the department they were met by a staff nurse who volunteered to accompany the group to the ward. Throughout the journey, during which time she looked at or spoke to Tommy only once, when Jenny asked him if he was all right, the staff nurse kept up a constant criticism, addressed to the porter, of the sister on duty that night and her apparent incompetence and unwillingness to do her work. As they entered the ward the staff nurse indicated an area where Tommy's relatives were to wait and Tommy was taken into the ward. Jim and Jenny were worried to think that the ward was in the charge of a sister who, according to the staff nurse, was so incompetent.

Jenny passed the next few minutes reading the literature that was pinned to the walls of the area in which they waited. One notice declared that a self-care nursing model was in use in that ward.

After a short time, a young nurse appeared. She had a badge identifying her as a student nurse and two stripes on her shoulder epaulettes. She explained that she needed some details and began to go through 'name, date of birth, address and type of accommodation'. The student then said that Jim and Jenny could go in and see Tommy and they realised that no questions had been asked about Tommy's many problems, with which they were very familiar. He was completely deaf and the only way to get through to him was to stand in front of him and shout so that he could pick up a few sounds to add to his limited ability to lip-read. Jenny told the nurse this, and that Tommy's present confused state would make things worse, but the nurse didn't write it down, just gave a little giggle and said: 'Oh, dear'.

They followed her along the corridor, past two staff nurses talking at the nurses' station, until she said: 'He's in there, behind the curtains.' So he was, unable to remember how he had got there or why. Jim explained and said they would come back in the morning with Tommy's wife. On the way out they stopped to ask the staff nurses if that would be all right. Neither of them made any move to reply until Jenny repeated the question, and then one said: 'Yes.' That was the sole contact Jenny and Jim had with any trained nurse in the ward on Tommy's admission, although they had both expected to be given some idea of when Tommy might be seen by the hospital doctor and what might be done to help him, and to receive some reassurance.

In the morning the family popped back in to see Tommy who by then had stopped vomiting and was no longer confused. He was, however, very tired so they left him with the promise that they would return in the evening. When they did so it was to find that Tommy had been moved to another bay and that he was sitting up in bed complaining that he had not had his insulin or his supper. To begin with, the family thought that he was still a bit confused, but careful questioning supported his worries and, as it was now half past seven and Tommy said he was feeling as if he had a 'hypo' coming on, Jenny approached the sister.

cont ...

... cont

Tommy was right. He hadn't had anything to eat since his lunch at midday and his evening insulin had also been forgotten. When the sister asked the auxiliary why Tommy had not been given his supper, she said that she had taken it to the bay where Tommy had previously been. When she found he was not there she had come to the entrance of his present bay and shouted. When nobody replied, she took his supper away.

Five minutes later, Sister gave Tommy his insulin and the same auxiliary brought his supper, a triangular sealed packet of cheese and tomato sandwiches. There was no plate and when Tommy tried to open the packet the grated cheese and slices of tomato flew everywhere. At this Jenny and Jim had had enough. They asked to see the sister and told her exactly what they thought about the 'nursing care' in the hospital. The sister agreed that there had been very inadequate care and apologised profusely, promising that things would improve. The next day the family, with great relief, took Tommy home. As they left the ward they passed the 'self-care model' poster again. Jenny felt that the family's need to protect Tommy by watching every move the staff made gave the 'self-care' model a whole new meaning!

FEEDBACK: BREAKING THE CODE

Unfortunately, that story is true in all essentials. The registered nurses broke the code of conduct in the following ways:

- The sister and staff nurse in the accident and emergency department must have known about the sheet of ice outside the door but did nothing to protect patients or other staff from injury (Point 10 of the code)

- The two staff nurses in the ward where Tommy was admitted allowed a student nurse to carry out the first nursing interview, at which vital information about a patient is obtained and on which a significant part of a nursing diagnosis depends. As a result, no note was made of the fact that Tommy had great difficulty in communicating and, had his visitors not queried it, he could have spent nearly 20 hours without insulin or food because he didn't hear the auxiliary shouting his name (Point 2). Allowing a student nurse to carry out the nursing admission without supervision was certainly not assisting her to develop professional competence (Point 12)

- The ward sister allowed this elderly diabetic with peripheral neuropathy and poor eyesight to struggle with no plate for his food and agreed that there were, in fact, no plates of any sort in the ward, this being 'hospital policy'. This is a clear example of lack of resources to which she should previously have drawn the attention of her line manager (Point 10)

- The ward sister failed to ensure that this patient received his insulin and his food (Point 2)

- All three of the staff nurses on night duty, and the ward sister as well, failed overall in their obligation to justify public trust and to safeguard the interests of the patient.

Did your answers to Activity 10 identify these points? Rethink the advantages of registration you identified in Activity 6. Can you identify any further advantages to having a legal system of registration of nurses that you would now add to your original list?

One thing that really needs emphasising is the fact that as registered nurses we are *all* accountable for our own actions. Accountability means that we are each responsible for what we do as professionals.

P4(ii): The competences in context looks in detail at the level-1 competences towards which you are now working, and considers the limitations and responsibilities of the first-level nurse. The discussion of nursing ideologies at the beginning of this Part is then linked to nursing philosophies and the use of the nursing process and nursing models. In the meantime, continue to reflect on the UKCC *Code of Professional Conduct* and its relevance to your present work. You are probably familiar with this brief statement from the code:

'Each registered nurse, midwife and health visitor shall act, at all times, in such a manner as to:

- Safeguard and promote the interests of individuals and clients

- Serve the interests of society

- Justify public trust and confidence

- Uphold and enhance the good standing and reputation of the professions'[8].

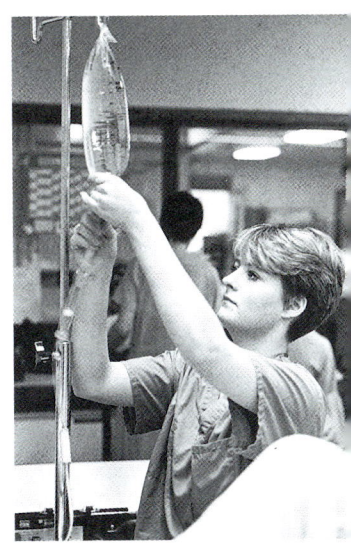

FOCUS

Absolutely for your diary only. Consider your own achievement of the UKCC *Code of Professional Conduct* principles by thinking back over the past six months or so. Go through the points in the Code and search your mind for any occasions when you might have broken it. Note them down, detailing what happened, why you think the circumstances came about and what you think you should have done. If there is still any action that you ought to take, put in a written report now! Can you identify any further advantages to having a legal system of registration of nurses that you would now add to your original list?

REFERENCES

1 Fuller, T. Exanthomatologia; A rational account of eruptive fevers. In: Austin, A. *History of Nursing Source Book*. New York: G.P. Putnam's Sons, 1957.

2 UKCC. *Project 2000. Project Paper 9. The final proposals*. London: UKCC, 1987.

3 Nurses Registration Act 1919. London: HMSO, 1919.

4 Bedford Fenwick, E.G. *The British Journal of Nursing* 1919; LXIII,1631 (editorial).

5 Nurses, Midwives and Health Visitors Act 1979. London: HMSO, 1979.

6 European Community Council Directive (77/453/EEC). Luxembourg: European Community, 1977.

7 *Nurses, Midwives and Health Visitors Rules Approval Order 1983*. London: HMSO, 1983.

8 UKCC. *Code of Professional Conduct for the Nurse, Midwife and Health Visito.* (3rd edn). London: UKCC, 1992.

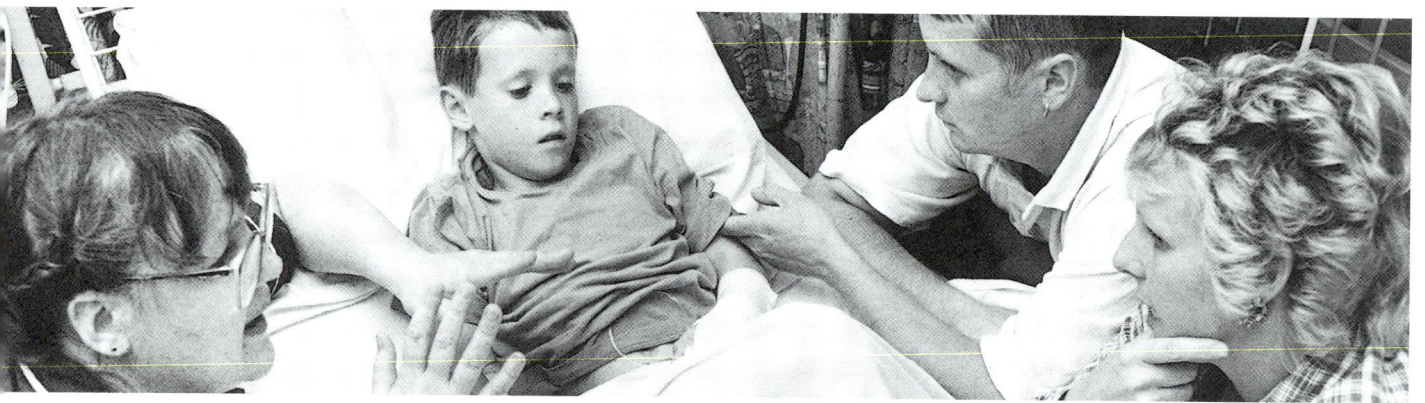

The competences in context

The Nurses, Midwives and Health Visitors Rules Approval Order 1983 lays down competences that every registered nurse must meet. In this Part you will look at:

- The three key areas of a level-1 nurse's role

- Accountability

- Nursing philosophies

- Before and after the nursing process

- Nursing models

- Conceptualised learning and becoming a 'knowledgeable doer'.

WORK PLANNER

You will need to refer back, if you have completed it, to the work you did in *P4(i): 'What is a registered nurse?'* where the level-2 and level-1 competences are listed.

THE THREE KEY AREAS

P4(i): What is a registered nurse? considered the factors that combine to make a registered nurse. It looked briefly at the *nursing competences* which are a legal requirement that every registered nurse must meet. The competences required to register as a level-1 nurse are different from those necessary for registration at level 2.

ACTIVITY 1
action
If you have worked through *P4(i) What is a registered nurse?* look back over the work you did. In Activity 7, you identified the differences between the competences you have been required to meet as an enrolled nurse and those you need to acquire to become a level-1 registered nurse. If you have your answers to that Activity to hand, check them off with the list alongside.

The differences are that:

- You will have a responsibility for advising on the promotion of health and the prevention of illness

- You will have to have the knowledge and skills necessary to advise on situations that may be detrimental to health and well-being

- You will need to be able to assess nursing requirements, make and implement a nursing care plan, teach and manage others who are involved in the plan, and review the effectiveness of the nursing care being given. (These activities form the 'nursing process', which we will be look at in more detail later.)

- You will develop the knowledge and skills involved in managing the care of a group of patients over a period of time.

It has long been recognised that enrolled nurses are often called upon to undertake level-1 roles. Many of you, therefore, have already achieved at least some of the level-1 competences, which should have been recognised in the profile you drew up at the start of the programme. We can simplify the differences listed above into three key areas in which, during this programme, you will be developing your knowledge, skills and responsibilities.

These three areas are:

- Health promotion

- The nursing process

- Personal, and that may mean sole, responsibility for all aspects of nursing care.

These are large parts of a level-1 nurse's role. Other parts of this course look at different ideas of health and illness, and consider health promotion, the nursing process and the use of nursing models. Throughout this programme, we keep focusing on the themes of reflective practice, self-awareness and working constructively as a member of the many groups of which you may form a part. These themes add up to the development of the 'knowledgeable doer', described in Project 2000 as one who accepts personal responsibility for professional actions.

ACCOUNTABILITY

The nursing competences for a level-1 nurse mean that we are all responsible for our own actions and we cannot blame anyone else if we do not meet the specified levels of competence. This personal responsibility is known as *accountability* — taking responsibility for our own actions. Registered nurses are solely accountable for their own actions. In addition, it must follow that level-1 registered nurses are accountable for the actions of those who give care under their direction if it can be shown that their direction or supervision were negligent. However, even though registered nurses are accountable for their own actions, they work in a society and with many professional colleagues who exert great influence on their role.

NURSING PHILOSOPHIES

Our discussion in *P4(i): What is a registered nurse?* uses the word ideology to mean 'a set of ideas that reflect the beliefs and interests of a group with a common purpose'.

There is a subtle difference between an ideology and what an individual thinks about the same subject.

ACTIVITY 2
diary
Write down, in two or three sentences if possible, what you think nursing 'is'. Start off by using the words:
'I believe nursing is ... '

You have just written your own personal nursing *philosophy*. A philosophy can be defined as 'a study of the basic principles and concepts of a discipline', as 'a system of beliefs or values' and as 'a personal outlook or viewpoint'. These all add up to a personal view about what, in that person's opinion, something should be. A nursing philosophy can therefore be described as a personal definition of nursing, such as you wrote in Activity 2.

There has long been a debate over whether nursing is an *art*, a *science*, or a bit of both. The Greek philosopher Aristotle said that 'science consists of things that are known and cannot be any different from the way they are'[1].

EXAMPLE

In nursing, we know scientifically that if a person remains lying or sitting in one position for a prolonged period of time, pressure sores will develop. Additionally, we know scientifically that several other factors also predispose to the development of pressure sores.

Art, as Aristotle describes it, is a *technical skill*. He says that every art is concerned with bringing something into being and that the practice of an art is the study of how to do that.

EXAMPLE

Continuing with our example of preventing the development of pressure sores, the art of nursing lies in the technical skills of giving each individual the care required to prevent the development of pressure sores. In this example, therefore, we have combined the use of scientific knowledge that pressure sores will develop in particular circumstances, with the art of using appropriate nursing skills to prevent this happening. If you look carefully at nursing philosophies you will find that most of them combine both science and art.

Let's look now at some other people's philosophies of nursing.

One of the best known nursing philosophies is that of Virginia Henderson[2]:

'The unique function of the nurse is to assist the individual, sick or well, in performance of those activities contributing to health or its recovery (or to a peaceful death) that he/she would perform unaided if he/she had the necessary strength, will or knowledge. And to do this in such a way as to help him/her gain independence as rapidly as possible.'

Now have a look at this alternative[3]:

- 'Nursing is caring, a quality that has been characteristic of nursing since its inception. It continues to be guarded fervently

- Nursing involves close personal contact with the recipient of care

- Nursing is concerned with services that take humans into account as physiological, psychological and sociological organisms

- Nursing is committed to personalised services for all persons without regard to colour, creed or social or economic status

- Nursing is committed to promoting individual, family, community and national health goals in the best manner possible

- Nursing is committed to involvement in ethical, legal and political issues in the delivery of health care'.

That philosophy is presented by its authors as a set of 'characteristics of nursing today'; but, in fact, it is a very comprehensive philosophy, including clear descriptions of the parts played by science and art.

It is no easy task for any of us to decide exactly what we personally think nursing should be. Generally speaking, most of us were told what someone else thought when we entered nurse training and, because they were frequently much older and had been nursing for a considerable period, we probably didn't question it much. Now, have another think about what you wrote in Activity 2: your own philosophy of nursing.

ACTIVITY 3
diary
Would you now add to, or alter, your own philosophy of nursing in any way? If so, rewrite it now. Can you see either science or art, or both, in it?

Of course, many of us share very similar philosophies. Because that described by Virginia Henderson is considered by many people to describe exactly how they also feel about 'what nursing should be', it is often adopted as the overall philosophy of individual colleges of nursing

THE NURSING PROCESS

ACTIVITY 4
diary
Has your college of nursing adopted a particular nursing philosophy? Make a note of it and then consider if you agree with it or if there are any alterations you would make. Write down your reasons. How does this philosophy differ from your own?

Whatever your philosophy of care, you need a way of organising it efficiently and appropriately for each individual. If you look at the competences of a level-1 nurse in *P4(i): What is a registered nurse?* you will see that (c) to (g) are a pretty clear description of the nursing process. However, by not naming the nursing process, the competences do leave room for other methods of individualised care to be evolved and adopted.

It has been pointed out that the nursing process is nothing new[4].

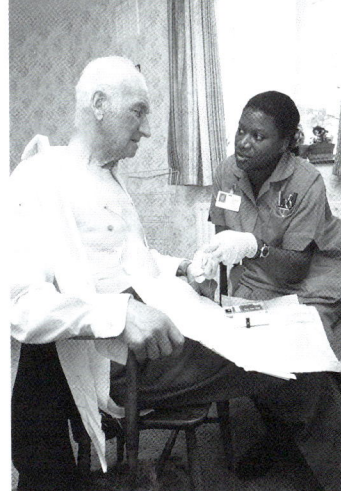

ACTIVITY 5
action
Ask any nurse who qualified before 1970 to describe how nursing care was (1) decided upon, (2) planned, (3) given and (4) judged for effectiveness, before the nursing process was used. Try to use those four headings. If you qualified before that time you can consider this from personal experience.

FEEDBACK

The nursing process has four stages which can be matched with the four headings you have just used:

1. Identifying what nursing needs each individual person has (*assessment*)

2. Planning nursing care designed specifically to meet the identified nursing needs (*planning*)

3. Seeing that each person is actually given the nursing care that has been decided upon, and to an adequate standard (*implementation*)

4. Judging whether the care given has been effective in meeting the nursing needs (*evaluation*).

The process is continuous. Evaluation and reassessment need to start with implementation, because nursing needs can alter very quickly and, additionally, it can rapidly become apparent that planned care is not having the desired effect and that a different approach is required.

ACTIVITY 6
diary
Consider your answers in the previous Activity. What are the main differences in the way nursing care was managed before and since the use of the nursing process?

FEEDBACK

The differences that most people identify are that before the use of the nursing process nurses did not usually work systematically through the different stages. Additionally, much of the process went on in their heads. That meant that a nurse used some personal method of working out what a patient's nursing needs were.

Notes

ACTIVITY 7
diary
Look back to Activity 5. Under 'describing how nursing care was decided upon', can you identify which member of staff generally 'prescribed' the nursing care? Is there any clue as to how that person worked out what a patient's nursing needs were?

FEEDBACK

Before the use of the nursing process, although there might well have been several qualified nurses in a department or ward, the nursing care for all patients was usually decided upon by the most senior in rank among them. This was invariably the sister or charge nurse and the care was frequently decided upon by looking at the patient's medical diagnosis.

EXAMPLE

All '1st day post-operative appendectomies' were given limited fluids, had a bed-bath in the morning and were sat out of bed for one hour. It didn't matter if they had only returned from theatre at five minutes to midnight, they were 'first day post-op' and that was that! This sort of nursing did not take any account of individual needs and did not take the whole person into consideration because it was not based on any model of care which helped identify specific requirements.

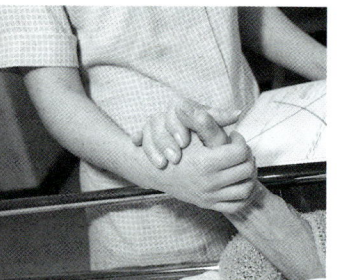

NURSING MODELS

The relationship of nursing models to the nursing process is very simple. If you are going to use a system of individualised care, which is what the nursing process is, you need some relatively foolproof way to help you look at each individual and identify nursing needs. Such a way of looking at an individual should also help you to plan and implement care appropriately and carry out effective evaluation. Different models are simply different ways of looking at an individual — nothing more complicated than that. We look at some of the most widely used nursing models in *P11: Models for Care*.

Figure 1 illustrates the simple relationship between the very important concepts we have discussed.

Fig. 1. Ways of achieving individualised care

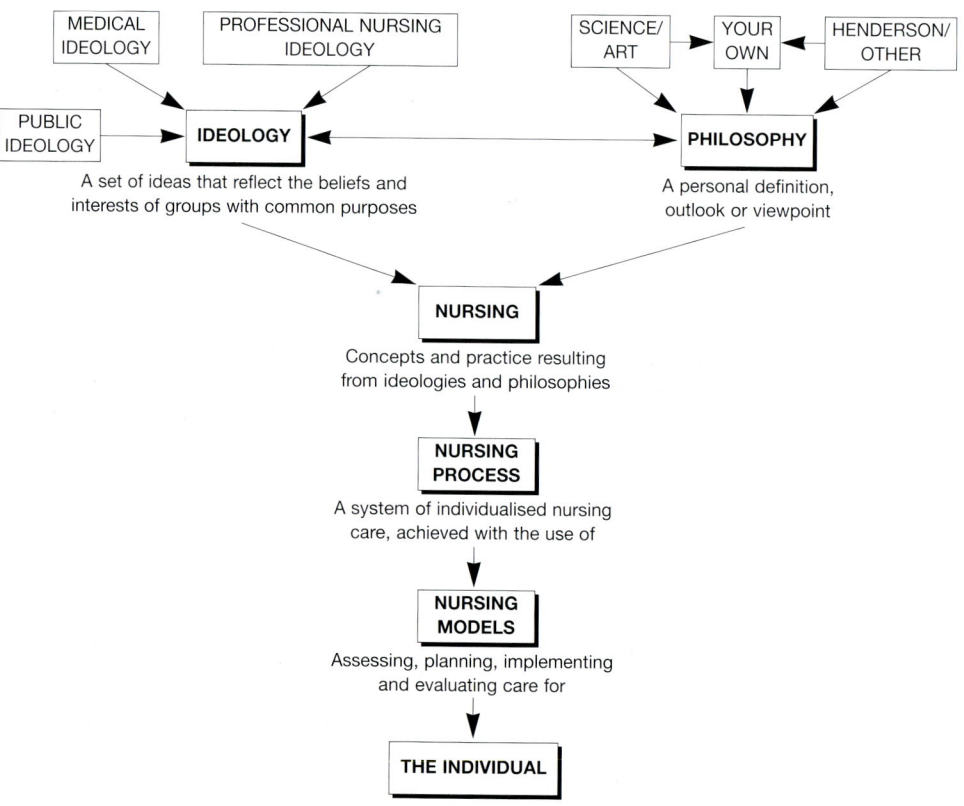

Notes

At this point it would be useful to come back to the concept of evidence-based practice (EBP) which was first summarised in *R1: Nursing: A Research-based Profession*. Read the following definition:

> 'It [EBP] involves identifying the problem, asking questions, searching the literature for answers and then deciding what intervention to adopt for that problem, based on the evidence available'[5].

Finally, we should look at the ways in which the new 'knowledgeable doer' needs to develop broader and deeper thinking about nursing.

CONCEPTUALISING

A concept is a general idea. In nursing practice we often use concepts, although we may not be aware that we are doing so. We have just been discussing one of them, the concept of individualised care — the idea of each individual patient having nursing care specifically planned, given and evaluated according to carefully identified nursing needs. *Conceptualising* means the act of forming a concept, getting a broad and useful idea together. Nursing concepts are all to do with thinking in an intelligent and constructive way.

Because nurse education now prepares people to become 'knowledgeable doers', it is very much centred on conceptualised learning. This means that students are no longer taught lists of items that should or should not be ticked off, carried out or attended to, but are taught to consider a whole range of information, possible courses of actions and their results, and to make appropriate choices in each individual situation. This programme is intended to give you every opportunity that we can offer to form meaningful and useful nursing concepts, instead of being told what you should think and do. The benefit of conceptualised learning is that it forces us all to argue the 'fors' and 'againsts' of every subject and action. However, skills remain of equal importance, hence the word 'doer' linked to the word 'knowledgeable'.

The following extract from the Emap Healthcare Open Learning mission statement sums up key aspects of learning to become a 'knowledgeable doer':

- To become autonomous practitioners, professionals need to be self-directed

- A programme of learning should focus on the learning process rather than on factual content

- The key to learning how to learn is through inquiry, reflection, evaluation and action

- Practice-based learning is the stimulus for raising standards of care generally.

P4(iii): Acquiring level-1 competences examines each of the level-1 competences in more detail.

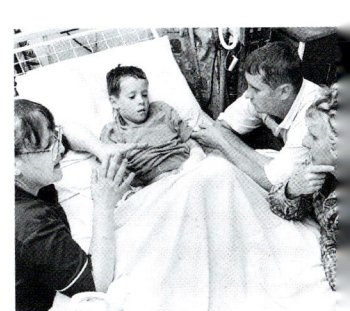

FOCUS

Think about what you have understood so far about being a level-1 nurse and the nursing process. Write a short paragraph describing these. You may find it helpful to look back through this Part and pick out words and phrases to use, such as 'individualised care' and 'accountability'.

REFERENCES

1 Aristotle. *The Nicomachean Ethics*. (Thomson, J.A.K., trans; revised edn). London: Penguin Books, 1976.

2 Henderson, V. *Basic Principles of Nursing Care*. London: International Council of Nurses, 1960.

3 Wolff L., Wetzel M., Zorrow R., Zsobar, H. *Fundamentals of Nursing*. (7th edn). Philadelphia: J.B. Lippincott Company, 1983.

4 Roper, N., Logan, W., Tierney, A. *Learning to Use the Process of Nursing*. Edinburgh: Churchill Livingstone, 1981.

5 White, Suzanne, J. Evidence-based practice and nursing: The new panacea. *British Journal of Nursing* 1997; **6**: 3.

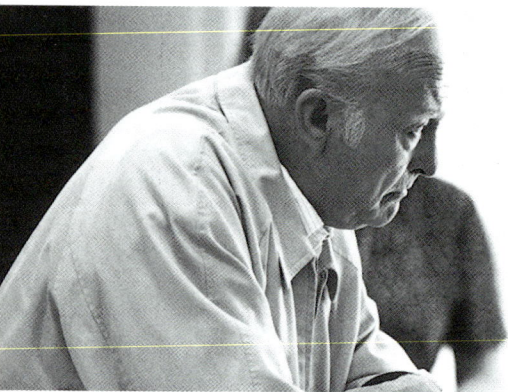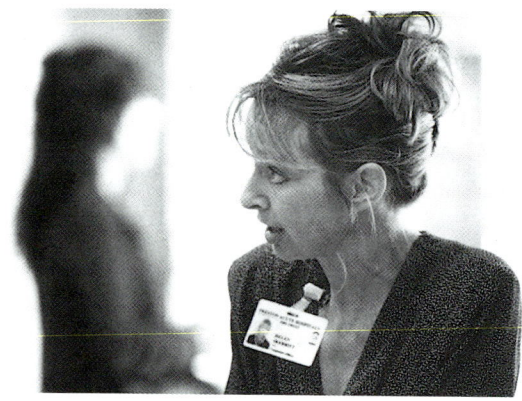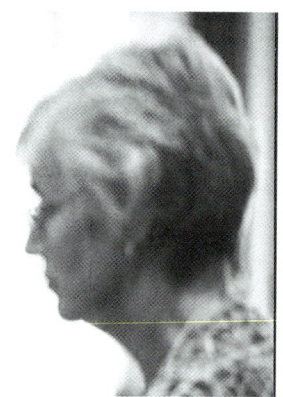

Acquiring level-1 competences

Parts (i) and (ii) of *P4: Nursing Competency*, looked at the general issues of the meaning and implications of nurse registration. In this Part you will look at how the level-1 competences relate to your own nursing knowledge and practice.

You will consider each of the competences in turn and think about the skills and knowledge you will need to meet these competences. As well as identifying your strengths, you will also be asked to pinpoint areas for development.

WORK PLANNER

There are several Activities here which ask you to reflect on your present level of competence. Although you may prefer to carry out much of this reflection privately, you may find it helpful, and reassuring, to seek the support of your clinical supervisor (mentor) or tutor/counsellor for some of these Activities.

Your clinical supervisor will be of particular help if you have trouble with Activity 9, which asks you to seek the opinion of colleagues on your effectiveness as a team member.

Activity 7 asks you to read a section of the document *The Scope of Professional Practice*, published by the UKCC in 1992. Your library should have a copy.

THE INDIVIDUAL COMPETENCES

We now go to your own field of nursing practice so that you can try to decide exactly how you, as an individual, need to develop in order to acquire level-1 competences. To do that we look at each of the competences in turn.

Health Promotion

(a) **advise on the promotion of health and the prevention of illness**

A report from King Edward's Hospital Fund for London[1] argued that health promotion:

'Implies two levels of action. At policy level it means laying the responsibility for promoting health on the government (and not just the Department of Health), public authorities and the various other agencies and interests which control, influence and fashion many of the basic features of our society. It implies a multi-sectoral collaboration to promote health. At community level it means enabling individuals and organisations to improve health through informed self-care, self-help and mutual aid.'

P1(i): A personal view of health and illness looked at some of the factors that influence the ideas an individual has about being 'well' or 'ill'. What about enabling individuals to improve health?

Health promotion is the subject of P7. It considers further the part that health promotion plays in your clinical practice.

(b) recognise situations that may be detrimental to the health and well-being of the individual

At first sight this competence appears fairly straightforward. In the discussion in *P4(i): What is a registered nurse?* of the ways in which a group of registered nurses failed to meet the UKCC *Code of Professional Conduct*, a situation where people were continually allowed to get out of ambulances and cars outside an A&E department onto a large sheet of ice was described. This was obviously detrimental to health! The same applies to allowing people to get out of bed onto a floor that is wet, or not reporting that a wire from a bedside nurse-call handset has become trapped in a bedside and stripped of its insulation covering.

However, there are deeper levels to this competence.

EXAMPLES

If you have a patient who is profoundly depressed you have a very clear responsibility to try to make some assessment of his/her potential for attempting suicide, and to act accordingly. Equally, if you become aware that a person is suffering a delusion that he or she is to attack anyone who approaches too closely, you have an obligation to act to protect others from harm. Consider this, possibly more common, example:

CASE STUDY

Gary Griffiths has been in your ward for some weeks following a motorbike accident. He has not found hospital food to his liking and his mother has regularly been bringing him sandwiches and cakes. At the weekend she brought him a large container which Gary put in his locker which was next to a radiator. You saw the container there and Gary told you what was in it but you didn't think twice about it. On Monday, thinking that the remaining sandwiches ought to be eaten up, Gary went round the ward offering them to the other patients for their teas. You thought it was very generous of him but by the next morning several patients were very ill and the laboratory reported that the ward was the site of a salmonella outbreak. You had failed to recognise a situation that might be detrimental to health.

Individualised Care

The next five competences require the level 1 nurse to give individualised care using a problem-solving approach. As explained in *P4(ii) The competences in context*, in practice at the moment this effectively means using the nursing process:

The first two of this group of competences relate to assessment:

(c) carry out those activities involved when conducting the comprehensive assessment of a person's nursing requirements

and

(d) recognise the significance of the observations made and use them to develop an initial nursing assessment

These two Activities should be undertaken when any individual needs nursing advice, support or care. They help you to understand, as much as possible, that each person is an individual, with individual relationships and living in an individual social setting. If you don't take these factors into consideration, the care that you plan and attempt to implement may be a disastrous failure.

EXAMPLES

In Helen Forrester's biography[2] she describes how, before the use of the nursing process, the school nurse instructed the family to buy lotion to put on the verminous heads of the children. The nurse's lack of understanding of the fact that the family had no money for food, let alone for lotion for treating head lice, meant that her 'nursing intervention' — the advice she gave — was totally useless.

Similarly, your advice to the parents of a 17-year-old boy with learning disabilities, to let him go into town alone to gain independence, may be inappropriate if you do not know that his recently developed habit of masturbating when in the company of other people has already resulted in problems.

ACTIVITY 3
diary
Describe the knowledge and skills you feel you will need to develop in order to meet the level-1 competences (c) and (d). Remember that your clinical supervisor (mentor) or tutor/counsellor will help to identify the areas of knowledge and skills you need to reach level 1 competences, if you feel you need some support in this.

The assessment of needs and the use of suitable and correctly made observations are the foundation of the nursing process. Without a sound foundation, your planning and implementation may be totally inappropriate.

Confidentiality. As soon as you come into contact with a patient, you are in possession of confidential information — the fact that the person is receiving nursing care. The carrying out of assessment and observation as part of the nursing process effectively means that you are in possession of many very personal details. People allow us, as nurses, to have such information because they trust us to use it for their good. In doing so they expect us, and we are obliged by the UKCC *Code of Professional Conduct*[3], to keep that information totally confidential. Maintaining confidentiality has become a problem and it is easy to think that those most likely to breach confidentiality would be relatively untrained health care assistants or new students, but this is not necessarily so.

CASE STUDY

Joan is a nurse consultant specialising in the care of people with a fairly common condition. When interviewing a new client, Frank, a few years ago, she discovered that he had been a fireman. Without stopping to think she said:

'Oh, I've got another client who was a fireman, Jim MacClain, do you know him?'

Frank said that he did, and expressed his surprise that Jim had 'got what I've got'.

That was Joan's first mistake, for she had no right to disclose the confidential information that Jim was a patient of hers, or of anybody else for that matter. Whenever Frank saw Joan after that he asked after Jim. On the last occasion Joan said:

'Oh, it's very sad, he's dying. Cancer, I'm afraid. There's nothing they can do.'

Frank was very upset and decided to get in touch with Jim's wife. When he did so it became clear that Jim did not know that he was dying and had obviously not given Joan permission to give anyone any information about him. Frank began to worry about what she might be saying to other people about him and made sure that in future he kept his worries about his health to himself.

Joan was in clear breach of the UKCC *Code of Professional Conduct*. Had anyone complained, she could have been disciplined. Additionally, and this is an important part of the reasoning behind the Code, Joan had lost the trust of her client. All the information we as nurses have about our patients, however trivial and apparently harmless, such as the sort of house a person lives in and whether he or she is married or not, is confidential.

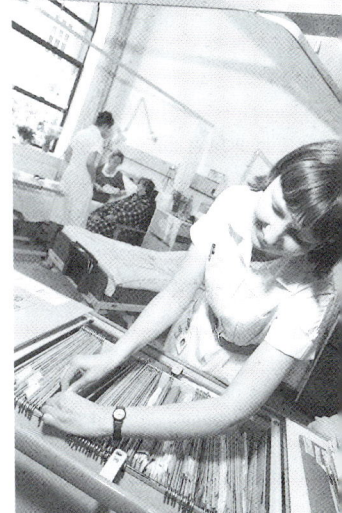

ACTIVITY 4
diary
Think carefully through the subject of confidentiality and, for your diary's eyes only, note down any areas where you think you personally need to take more care not to reveal confidential information.

(e) **devise a plan of nursing care based on the assessment with the co-operation of the patient, to the extent that this is possible, taking into account the medical prescription**

This competence calls for a very high level of nursing knowledge and skills. You need to know the complete range of possible courses of action and be able to judge why each is more or less appropriate in the particular situation. You also need the skills of discussing the choices with the patient where possible. Many older people expect a nurse to 'tell them what is going to be done for them', rather than discuss what action the patient would prefer and the parts the nurse and patient will each play in that. Clearly, then, the selection of choices of care and the planning that results are critical parts of the process. How this part of the nursing process is actually carried out will be discussed in a later Section. What you need to do now is to look at your present understanding of the planning process and identify exactly where you need to develop.

ACTIVITY 5
diary
Work out and note down the knowledge and skills you think you need to acquire in the next few months in relation to the planning of care.

(f) **implement the planned programme of nursing care and, where appropriate, teach and co-ordinate other members of the caring team who may be responsible for implementing specific aspects of the nursing care**

In plain terms, 'implementing' care means 'giving' care in a satisfactory way, and in this case seeing that others who give care do so to an adequate standard. This means that we must teach others who do not have the necessary knowledge and skills, whether they are care assistants, students or other qualified colleagues. There has now been a great deal of work done on setting simple and effective standards of care, but this will not help if each individual nurse does not have the required knowledge and skills to achieve them.

EXAMPLE

Suppose that your community area or ward has a standard of care in relation to patients with urinary catheters. Perhaps it is worded as follows:

'Patients with indwelling urinary catheters will remain free from urinary infection.'

That is certainly acceptable because urinary infections, besides causing considerable pain and discomfort, can result in very serious problems. The standard is achievable if everyone concerned gives adequate catheter care. It is observable because we can tell whether a patient remains free of urinary infection and it is measurable because we can count what percentage of catheterised patients remain infection-free. However, problems can still arise. Read the following case study to see what can happen.

CASE STUDY

Night duty as a relief staff nurse is not an easy life, but **Mandy** likes the varied work and the new challenges that she meets. On one spell of duty, however, she came across a problem that really set her back. She was sent to relieve the night sister in a part of the hospital in which she had not previously worked, while the sister took her break. As she went round Mandy noticed that all the urinary drainage bags were off their holders and lying on the floor. Thinking that a new care assistant had done this, Mandy put matters to rights. When the sister returned she took one look and said: 'Who put those bags back on their holders?' Mandy explained, only to be told that, in the sister's opinion, 'they drained better if the bags were on the floor'. Mandy pointed out that there was a terrible risk of contamination from dust and said that it really worried her, but the sister would not listen and went round putting the bags back on the floor.

Mandy realised that she needed some sound information and evidence to challenge the sister's argument. She also realised that discussing the problem with other staff, without the sister's involvement, could be considered unprofessional although she wanted to resolve the problem as soon as possible.

The next day, as soon as she got up, Mandy went to her professional library. There she searched through books and journals until she came to a research-based article that quite clearly stated that contamination of drainage bags by contact with floors or other potentially soiled surfaces must be avoided at all costs. Mandy took details of the appropriate article and, that night, asked to talk to the sister in private. When confronted with the evidence that what she had been doing was incorrect, the sister agreed to follow the advice of the article and always keep the drainage bags suspended clear of the floor. Additionally, she asked Mandy if she would be prepared to produce a reading list on the care of catheterised patients for use by all night staff. Mandy agreed. She had not found taking action easy — in fact it had been very stressful — but she had an obligation as a registered nurse to do so. In fact, in this instance, she had also had to 'teach' another member of the caring team who was a higher grade than herself.

ACTIVITY 6
diary
Is your clinical knowledge adequate? Do you honestly always know what you are doing? Is your clinical care based on sound knowledge? Again, just between you and your diary, identify any areas of clinical knowledge or skill which you are not really sure of, or where you now think you may be out of date. Make a note of the action you will take to fill in the gaps in your knowledge and bring yourself up to date.

Competence (f) presents us with an additional problem. Nursing care is constantly changing and nurses are asked, or sometimes simply expected, to take on roles that they have not previously fulfilled. Until recently this was known as the 'extended role' of the nurse, a role for which different authorities and institutions had different policies relating to training and assessing competence. This often meant that anyone changing jobs might have to undergo the same training and assessment process again for the new authority.

The UKCC guidelines, included in the document *The Scope of Professional Practice*[4], have now set out a different approach to these additional elements of the nurse's role. These guidelines emphasise the individual nurse's professional accountability, and place decisions about the boundaries of practice in the hands of the individual practitioner[5]. Paragraph 9 of this document lays down six principles to help practitioners make these decisions about whether they are competent to carry out any additional aspects of care, and how to organise the necessary training through clinical nurse specialists.

ACTIVITY 7
knowledge base
Get hold of a copy of the UKCC document *The Scope of Professional Practice*. Read through the six principles in Paragraph 9, and use them as guidelines to identify any areas where you think you might need additional support (beyond the scope of this programme) to meet the demands made on your role.

(g) review the effectiveness of the nursing care provided and, where appropriate, initiate any action that may be required

Evaluation is, again, a major part of nursing care. It is no good making a nursing care plan and implementing it and then sitting back and letting it all happen! What happens may include complications that you hadn't even considered. Evaluation means constantly checking to see that the planned care is doing what it was intended to do and that new problems, either related to it or entirely unconnected, are not arising. At the moment you are expected to 'assist in reviewing the effectiveness of the care provided'. How good are you at this?

ACTIVITY 8
diary
Note down in your diary any aspects of evaluation of care that you want to learn more about. We shall be asking you to refer back to your notes when you study the nursing process in detail later on in the programme.

Teamwork

(h) work in a team with other nurses, and with medical and paramedical staff and social workers

You are already required to meet this competence. How well are you doing?

ACTIVITY 9
diary

Consider how well you work as a member of a team. If you feel that you can cope with possible criticism, write an honest account of how you feel you work in a team. Write down both your strengths and your weak points. Ask work colleagues both in nursing and other disciplines to comment, anonymously, on what you have written. Do they agree with your assessment of yourself? What else could they add?
It can be painful to receive adverse comments, especially anonymous ones. But the aim of this exercise is to help you to improve your performance (not to upset you). You may find it helpful to discuss the comments with your practice supervisor and decide on a few simple actions to improve your part in teamwork.

Managing Care

(i) undertake the management of the care of a group of patients over a period of time and organise the appropriate support services

This will officially be a new role for you. The management of a case-load, the care of a group of patients as a primary nurse or of a larger number of clients as a staff nurse in, for example, the community, will require some additional management skills.

ACTIVITY 10
diary

Note down the additional skills that you think you will need to take on the responsibility described in level-1 competence (i).

THE LEVEL-1 NURSE

P4(i): What is a registered nurse? described the terrible, though true, tale of Tommy whose 'nursing care' included the trained nurses forgetting his insulin and not ensuring that he had had his supper. The sequel to this story is also true in all essentials.

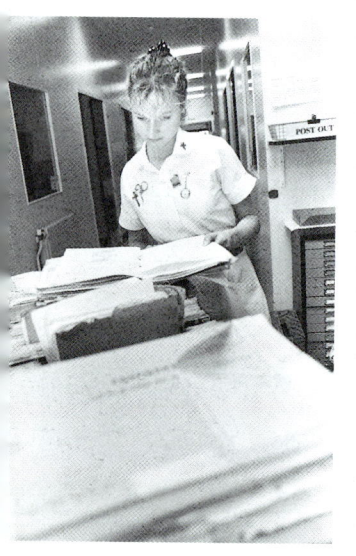

A few months after that incident, Tommy's wife, **Betty**, was out shopping when she fell over and suffered a fractured neck of femur and a Colles' fracture. After she was admitted to hospital, her first words to her daughter-in-law, Jenny, were: 'Oh goodness, fancy having to come to this place. Remember what they did to Tommy.'

However, things were so different that all the family were amazed. The charge nurse met Jenny as she came into the department and explained what had happened, what Betty's possible injuries were, and what would happen next. When it was realised that Betty had an 83-year-old husband for whom she usually cared, a social worker arrived to see if there was any immediate help that the family needed in looking after him. The staff nurse in the department saw Jenny looking at the X-rays and included her in the discussion with the casualty officer on diagnosis and surgical treatment. She then brought an injection of pethidine for Betty and allowed time for it to take effect before correcting the external rotation of her leg and applying skin extensions. Finally, she applied a plaster of Paris back slab to Betty's wrist. At all times this very competent nurse explained clearly and simply what she was about to do, and why.

On arrival at the ward Betty was greeted by name by an enrolled nurse and lifted into a bed that had already had a special mattress put on it. After bringing Betty and Jenny a cup of tea the enrolled nurse sat down with them and, explaining why she needed to know the answers, quietly and simply asked Betty for information about her usual living habits 'so we know what to aim for in helping you to get better'. The staff nurse came and introduced herself and said: 'Now don't lie here and worry and wonder. We'll try and explain everything but if there is anything else you want to know, just ask.'

cont ...

... cont

The next day, after a visit from the physiotherapist, Betty had her operation. That evening, as Jenny was going into the ward, the staff nurse stopped in the corridor and said that she was just off for her supper but that Betty was fine and Sister would have a word with Jenny if there was anything she wanted to know. The excellent standard of communication and care continued, with physiotherapists and occupational therapists being involved in the very well-co-ordinated care that the staff provided.

What can we conclude from that 'other side of the coin' account? Here we had four more qualified nurses, this time all totally competent, yet all working in the same hospital as those whose appalling 'care' caused Tommy such problems and distress, and who broke the UKCC *Code of Professional Conduct* in a number of ways. The message has to be that it is no use blaming 'the system', the 'management' or anything else. We are all responsible for, and therefore accountable for, our actions.

If the care we give is inadequate, if we fail to meet the competences for our level of registration, or if we fail to keep to the UKCC *Code of Professional Conduct*, the fault lies with each individual. That is what being a registered nurse means.

FOCUS

From all the Activities in this Part, write a clear summary of the knowledge and skills you feel you need to develop to enable you to achieve the level-1 competences. If you are already registered on the programme, use this as an opportunity to review your goal plans, and discuss any changes you feel you would like to make with your tutor/counsellor.

REFERENCES

1   King Edward's Hospital Fund for London. *The Nation's Health. A strategy for the 1990s.* London: King Edward's Hospital Fund for London, 1988.

2   Forrester, H. *Twopence to Cross the Mersey.* Glasgow: William Collins Sons & Co., 1974.

3   UKCC. *Code of Professional Conduct for the Nurse, Midwife and Health Visitor.* London: UKCC, 1984.

4   UKCC. *The Scope of Professional Practice.* London: UKCC, 1992.

5   Holder, S. Expanding role (letter). *Nursing Standard.* 1989; **38**: 3, 52.

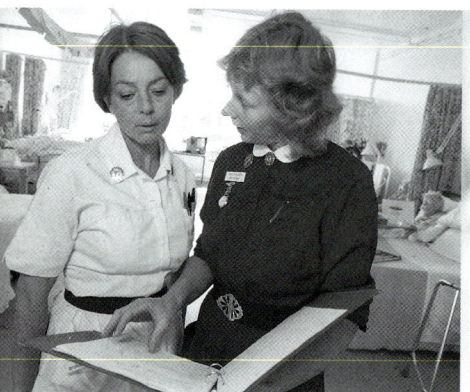
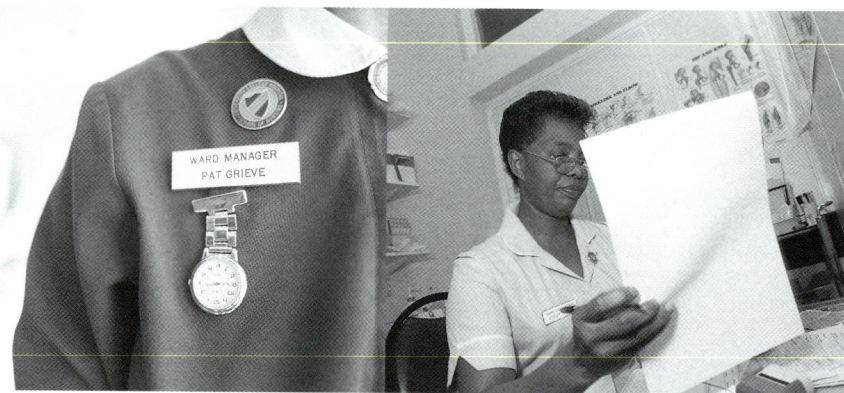

Are you a manager?

This first Part of *Principles of Management* considers what makes a manager and how managers work. You will:

- Draw up a definition of management

- Discover to what extent you are already a manager

- Look at the technical and managerial aspects of your job

- Look at the prescribed and discretionary aspects of your job

- Learn what it takes to make a good decision

- Focus on how to manage your time.

WORK PLANNER

Activity 2 asks you to look up a definition in a dictionary. Use the *Concise Oxford Dictionary* if you can.

As you work through this Section, you will find it helpful to have a copy of your job description to hand. You will also find it useful to refer to the 'Planning and observation' and 'Management skills' section of the Skills Inventory if you have worked through the Profile Pack.

The Focus asks you to compile a time log for a working week. It will be helpful, although not vital, if you can complete this log before moving on to *M1(ii): How do you manage?*

The following books are recommended further reading for *M1: Principles of Management*:

- Cole, G.A., *Management – Theory and Practice* (4th edn). London: Letts Educational Publishers, London, 1996.

- Mullins, L.J., *Management and Organisational Behaviour* (4th edn). London: Pitman Publishing, 1996.

- Weihrich, H., Koontz, H., *Management – A global perspective* (10th edn). New York: McGraw-Hill Inc., 1993.

WHAT IS MANAGEMENT?

ACTIVITY 1
diary
What do you think management is? Spend a few minutes making a list in your diary of the things managers do. Now think about your list in relation to your own workplace. Make a note of who 'does' each of the things on your list.

FEEDBACK

You might have listed activities such as 'being in charge', 'getting people to do things', 'making decisions', 'making forecasts and plans' and 'taking responsibility'.

Do you see management as something *you do*, or is it something other people do to you? Many enrolled nurses feel that they are already carrying out management activities which are not recognised or rewarded. We intend to explore this further in this Section.

Management of care is a key element in the level 1 competences. Throughout the Management module, we will be exploring the idea that we all need to manage, and that being a good manager has very little to do with what 'level' you are at in the healthcare hierarchy, or what specific type of professional training you have had.

The idea of management of healthcare resources is central to the changes taking place within the health service. Whether you work in the public or private sector, you will probably have met pressure to make more efficient use of resources — both human and financial — while maintaining care standards. You may have found this a difficult challenge to meet.

A good manager not only uses the resources available to her efficiently and effectively; she also does it with the support of those above her and below her in the hierarchy.

Like so many words in the English language, the words 'manage', 'management' and 'manager' have different meanings depending upon the context in which they are used, but many of the dictionary definitions are actually quite helpful.

WHAT DOES A MANAGER DO?

ACTIVITY 2
knowledge base
Look up the word 'manage' in a dictionary. We suggest you use the *Concise Oxford Dictionary*[1].
Make a list in your diary of words from the definitions which are relevant to your idea of management. Check this against your list in answer to Activity 1.

Henri Fayol[2], a French industrialist writing in the early part of this century, described the activities of managers under the six headings below:

- Forecasting
- Planning
- Organising
- Commanding
- Co-ordinating
- Controlling.

Although a variety of more complex descriptions have been developed since then, Fayol's elements of management are generally accepted as a good starting point for managers attempting to understand the nature of their role. However, one change of emphasis needs to be made to take account of the emergence of more enlightened approaches to management in modern work culture. The word *motivating* is more often used these days than *commanding*.

Notes

ACTIVITY 3
diary
How closely did the list of words you extracted from the dictionary definitions compare with Fayol's elements?

FEEDBACK

It's almost certain that you will have included 'organise' and 'control', although you may have used alternative words to describe the same ideas. The notion of *forecasting* and *planning* was probably implied by including in your list expressions such as 'succeed in one's aim', 'make proper use of' and 'administration'.

Co-ordinating suggests that managers are concerned with more than one activity or person, and your list may have included 'be manager of (team etc.)', 'controlling activities of person or team in sports, entertainment, etc.'

HOW DO MANAGERS MANAGE?

ACTIVITY 4
diary
Do any of the words used in the dictionary definitions above describe the behaviour of the managers you listed in answer to Activity 1?

FEEDBACK

You may have included in your list 'gain one's ends with (person etc.) by tact, flattery, dictation, etc.' This is particularly relevant when thinking about motivating: how we get others to perform according to our requirements.

Now is the moment to identify any elements of management in your own activities.

ACTIVITY 5
diary
Make a list in your diary of Fayol's six elements of management discussed above. Alongside each of these write down those activities from within your own job which seem to be described by that element. Use your job description, as well as thinking about what you actually do. Don't worry if you cannot find something to fit every element.

FEEDBACK

By now you may be discovering that there are elements of management in your own job. Many aspects of a nurse's work involve co-ordinating her skills with others to provide a service for patients. For example, if you work in a hospital you may co-ordinate the skills of other nurses and auxiliary staff.

ACTIVITY 6
diary
Read the following checklist and answer the questions to help you decide if you are already a manager.
• A manager works in an organisation (an organisation exists if people consciously combine their efforts for a common purpose). Do *you* work in an organisation? What is its common purpose?
• A manager is concerned with the efficiency of the organisation in seeing that it achieves its purpose. Are *you* in any way concerned with using resources in such a way as to make sure your organisation achieves its purpose efficiently?
• A manager's job is to see that the conditions are right for others to do their jobs effectively so that the purposes of the organisation can be achieved. Do *you* have any responsibility for providing the right conditions for other people to do their jobs effectively?

FEEDBACK

It would be surprising if you haven't answered 'yes' to at least one of these questions. You are more of a manager than you may have thought.

However, in common with most jobs, yours is unlikely to be totally concerned with management. Almost all jobs have both *technical* and *management* elements.

As the diagram below shows, the proportion of management content to technical content tends to increase as an individual rises in the organisation hierarchy.

MANAGEMENT LEVEL

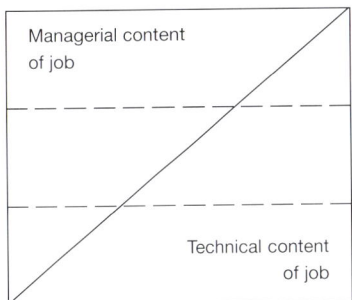

Senior

Middle

First-line

Notes

ACTIVITY 7
diary

In Activity 6 you identified those aspects of your job which could come under the heading 'management'. Now identify those aspects which could come under the heading 'technical'. Are there any aspects of your job which you cannot decide about? Do you want to add to your list of management activities?
As a result of this Activity you should now have a complete list of all your job activities.

FEEDBACK

It's quite easy to find examples from within healthcare of jobs which depend very heavily upon technical skill: pharmacist, surgeon, nurse, anaesthetist, laboratory technician, and so on. As we said earlier, it is not unusual for people holding positions with a high degree of technical content to assume that their jobs have little to do with management. But somebody has to manage, and if an organisation fails to achieve a balance between technical and management expertise the effects can be far-reaching.

EXAMPLE

The NHS has the technical capacity to offer ever more sophisticated operations and specialised treatments, yet the waiting lists for routine operations and treatment continue to grow.

ACTIVITY 8
diary

Identify some examples from your own experience of healthcare which show a similar imbalance between the technical and managerial content of jobs in the organisation. Can you identify, from Fayol's list, the elements of management which were not adequately covered?

WHAT MAKES AN EFFECTIVE MANAGER?

There are those who believe that good managers are born rather than made. While it is true that basic personality factors are important in management, there is also a lot of evidence to show that specific management skills can be learned. These skills will be major themes of the Management module, and we will be referring to them throughout.

Using Time

The activities which are crucial for successful management are not always the activities which take up most of our time. Effective time management is about identifying the importance of each individual activity, and allocating an appropriate amount of time to it.

There are various popular theories about the relationship between time, work and effectiveness. One of the most widely known is the Pareto effect, named after Vilfredo Pareto, who observed that 80% of our effectiveness comes from 20% of our activities. This observation led him to frame his 80/20 law which has been widely applied to many fields of human activity right up to the management of national economies.

Notes

Another theory comes from the popular post-war writings of Northcote Parkinson. One of the famous 'Parkinson's Laws' states that 'work expands to fit the time available'. This second 'law' has received support from the discovery that during the enforced three-day week crisis of the early seventies the nation achieved 80% of its normal output.

If there is anything to be learned from these 'laws' it seems to be that we are all likely to be in the position to make more effective use of our time. The extent to which we can do that depends upon identifying opportunities for becoming more effective. In the Focus Activity at the end of this Part you will have a chance to look in your own work environment for opportunities to become a better time manager.

Using Discretion

Earlier we made a distinction between the technical and management content of work and from Activities 7 and 8 you may have concluded that the technical aspects of work at your level in the organisation are often more significant than the management aspects. In terms of the proportion of the time you allocate to each aspect this is probably true.

However, we need to introduce another important dimension of management at this point — the amount of freedom (or *discretion*) an individual has to make decisions about a particular activity. The technical aspects of work are frequently *prescribed*, giving the individual little or no freedom to make decisions about how the work is done.

EXAMPLE

Procedures for the administering of medication (a technical aspect) are carefully prescribed to minimise the risk of error; while, in contrast, an individual nurse can exercise considerable discretion in how he or she communicates with patients when giving the medication.

It is unlikely that the prescribed and discretionary aspects of any job will coincide precisely with the technical and management aspects, but an appreciation of this distinction can help us to understand better our own management role.

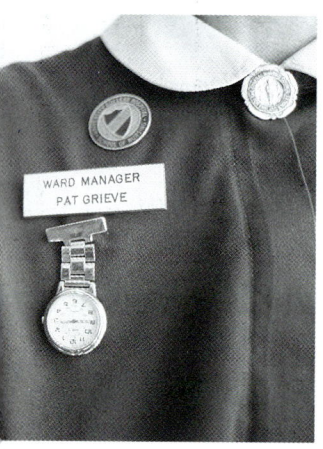

ACTIVITY 9
dairy
Look at your list of job activities from Activity 5. Make a note of the extent to which those activities are prescribed or discretionary. (Many activities have both prescribed and discretionary content — try to assess the proportion of each.)

FEEDBACK

Those aspects of your job which allow you to exercise discretion are likely to be the areas where there is most scope for improving your personal effectiveness, and therefore your skills of management.

Making Decisions

How well we exercise discretion depends upon our ability to make correct decisions. Decision-making is central to the role of any manager.

- To be effective a decision must have two characteristics: *quality* and *acceptance*.

  – A *good-quality* decision is one that provides the most economic outcome (that is, it makes the best use of scarce resources — money, people, facilities and equipment)

  – A decision has to be *accepted* by those who have to implement it, or these economic benefits will not be realised

- To make an effective decision we need to have sufficient information to take account of the feelings of those who have to work with the decision

- A problem arises when it is difficult to make a decision because there is insufficient information immediately available. Effective problem-solving is dependent upon our ability to:

  - gain access to the missing information, and/or

  - minimise the risk of making the wrong decision when a decision cannot be deferred

- The dilemma most of us face in taking decisions is finding a balance between speed and effectiveness: there is never sufficient time to find out everything we would like to know about a particular problem. One way out of this dilemma is to identify *priorities*. This process involves assessing the urgency and difficulty of each decision. Four categories of decision are probably sufficient:

  - Quick, get it out of the way first

  - Essential, take as long as it needs

  - Desirable, but could be deferred

  - Not urgent and not quick.

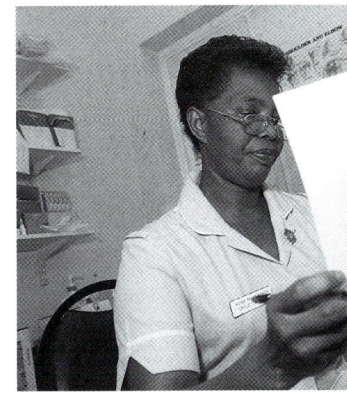

ACTIVITY 10
diary

Think of six decisions you have made recently in your everyday life (such as what to have for supper, where to go on holiday, how much you can afford to spend on a new bathroom suite), and at work. Can you allocate these to any of the above categories? Do you think you dealt with each decision in the most appropriate way? For example, did you make a snap decision about a holiday when you might have made a better decision if you had given it more thought, or did you spend so long thinking about something that events had overtaken you by the time you made the decision?

In *M1(ii): How do you manage?* we return to decision-making and look at the 'acceptance' part of making good management decisions. Acceptance is all about how the people you work with see you and your approach to management. We will also be exploring your own style of management, the 'people skills' which determine whether or not your decisions are effective.

The Focus asks you to do an exercise in managing your time more effectively.

FOCUS

This Activity asks you to consider how to use your time during work and leisure hours and to identify opportunities for becoming more effective in your use of time.

A good way of doing this is to keep a time log for two or three working days. Ideally, you should try to carry this out before starting work on *M1(ii): How do you manage?*

Start by creating a time log to cover each working day (see the example illustrated on page 126). Split your waking hours into half-hour slots, leaving sufficient space to record what you do. Make separate columns to record interruptions, and to make comments on the outcome of each activity.

There will probably be blocks of time that you can account for in advance, such as meal times and travelling times.

Complete the remainder of your log as frequently as time permits, ensuring that you record interruptions and their sources (for example, telephone, colleague).

When your log for each of the days is complete, you can set about the process of analysing how effectively you used your time. Here are some guidelines to help you with your analysis:

cont ...

... cont

Make brief notes in your diary in relation to each of these areas/questions:

- Add up the actual time taken up by interruptions

- Calculate how much time could have been saved by either refusing to be interrupted or curtailing the interruption

- Look carefully at time spent in meetings or discussion with colleagues and assess what these meetings and discussions actually achieved. Were the meetings necessary or too long relative to what they achieved?

- Would it have been possible to set aside periods of time to complete specific tasks rather than allow them to become fragmented or postponed?

Make a list showing the priority of the tasks which you completed during the time you logged, from most to least important, and calculate the time which you spent on each. Does the time allocation reflect the relative importance of the task?

Could the task have been rescheduled into a more logical sequence?

Identify the controlling factor for each task, for example, hospital routines, the work of others, and so on. Could any of these be changed?

Are you missing out on valuable leisure time by failing to manage time spent at work?

Conversely, are you allowing leisure to intrude upon your work?

Are you doing the work of others unnecessarily?

When your analysis is complete, use the time log format to draw up a revised schedule for a typical day showing the benefits in terms of time saved and more effective outcomes.

Sample Time Log

Day 1

Time Period	Activity	Interruptions	Comments/Outcomes
00.00 – 00.30			
00.30 – 01.00			
01.30 – 02.00			
02.00 – 02.30			
etc for 24 hours			

REFERENCES

1   *Concise Oxford Dictionary*, 9th edn. Oxford: Oxford University Press, 1995.
2   Fayol, H. *General and Industrial Management.* (Translated by Constance Storrs.) London: Pitman, 1949.

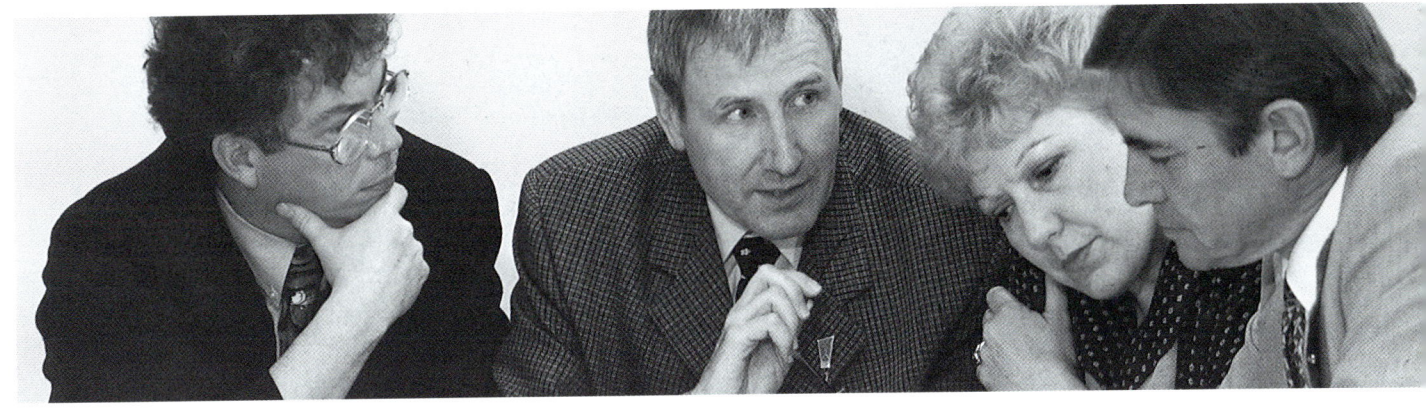

How do you manage?

The Focus in this Part is on identifying your own personal style of management and looking at the organisation for which you work.

You will consider:

- The balance between people and tasks
- Ways in which management styles change with different situations
- How management decisions are reached
- Task structure and position power within an organisation
- Interpersonal relationships — the key to successful management.

Notes

WORK PLANNER

In this Part you will reflect on your own management style, and the factors affecting management in your own organisation. You will find it helpful in doing this to identify someone with whom you can discuss these issues openly.

Activities 5, 8 and 15 are specifically flagged up for discussion. Your practice supervisor may well be the best person with whom to discuss your ideas, or you may prefer to identify another person in management. If you have problems in identifying a suitable person, contact your tutor/counsellor.

YOUR MANAGEMENT STYLE

A useful starting point for a discussion of management styles is to focus on the personality traits of the manager.

ACTIVITY 1
diary
Think about all the managers, good and bad, you have known.
Make some notes in your diary about the characteristics which made you categorise them as being 'good', 'bad' or somewhere in between.

FEEDBACK

The positive characteristics you noted may have included things like: 'considerate', 'good communicator', 'efficient', 'flexible', 'fair', 'consistent', 'supportive'. The direct opposites of these descriptions may appear in your list of unfavourable characteristics.

ACTIVITY 2
diary
Read through the problem that is printed alongside this Activity circle and list, in order of priority, the factors you would take into consideration in making the decision required. Note: You are not required to produce a duty rota.

You are responsible for a group of seven people, of whom three are of higher status in the organisation than the others. You are in the high-status group.

You are required to produce the annual holiday rota for the group, including yourself, not later than a month from now. The criteria are as follows:

- Everybody is entitled to four working weeks in addition to statutory national holidays, although those periods must be covered

- Normally, not more than three people can be on leave at the same time. However, between the beginning of October and the end of March the workload will not permit more than two people to be away from the department

- At least two weeks of the holiday entitlement must be taken as a block and it is not possible to carry holidays over into subsequent calendar years

- Of the group, including yourself, five are married and three are single. Four of the married people have children of school age.

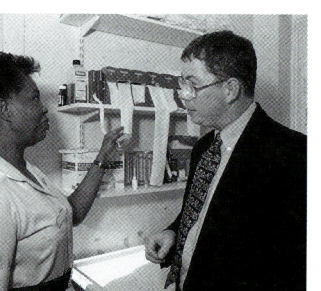

People and Tasks

A succession of social psychologists[1–3] have approached the question of what are appropriate qualities by looking at the manager's relative concern for *people* and *tasks*. Let's analyse your list of priorities in answer to Activity 2 using a similar approach to see if it can tell us anything about your style of management.

ACTIVITY 3
diary
Look at each item in your list from Activity 2 and assess whether it reflects a greater concern for tasks being completed or for people being satisfied. Mark task concerns with a 'T' and people concerns with a 'P'. A typical task concern would be, 'ensure that minimum staffing levels are maintained'; while a people concern would be: 'take account of school holidays for staff with children'.

FEEDBACK

The number of 'Ts' and 'Ps' in your list reflects your relative concern for tasks and people. Take particular note of the high-priority items in your list, as these are the best indicators of your management style. Most people show a bias towards either tasks or people, but very few people favour one to the total exclusion of the other.

The Activity which you have completed is only a rough guide to your style; a more detailed study would be capable of showing a more complete picture and it would be possible to plot your position on a matrix such as the one that appears below.

ACTIVITY 4
diary
Try to assess where your answer to Activity 3 places you on the matrix. Make a note in your diary.

Fig. 1. Matrix to assess relative concern for people and tasks

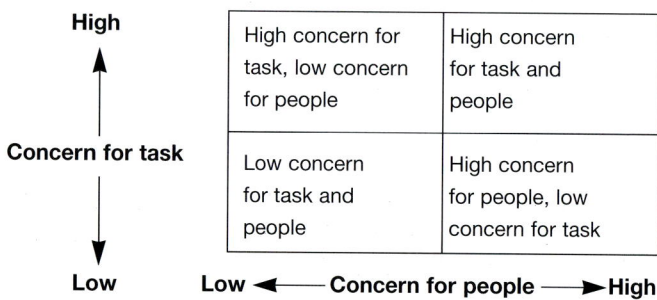

FEEDBACK

If you are in the top right quarter then you show a balanced concern for both people and task and your management style is conducive to high productivity and high morale.

If you have identified the upper left quarter, a high concern for task and low concern for people, then your management style is likely to ensure that tasks are completed ahead of schedule, but you are more likely to experience problems of low morale, and possibly suffer from higher than normal staff turnover, grievances and absenteeism.

The lower right quarter indicates a style which will probably create high morale, a warm and friendly environment, but with problems such as difficulty in the completion of tasks on schedule.

It is unlikely that you will have placed yourself in the bottom left corner. This indicates a style with low concern for both tasks and people, and anyone in this quarter probably isn't a manager at all!

In an ideal world, we would all be in the upper right quarter on the matrix, and one benefit of this approach to assessing management styles is that it gives an indication of the direction in which a manager needs to develop.

ACTIVITY 5
discussion
Depending on which quarter of the matrix you placed yourself in Activity 4, make a few notes on the areas you need to develop in your own management style. Discuss your notes with your practice supervisor or other mentor.

FEEDBACK

This Activity may have suggested that you need to develop more 'people' skills, or it may have suggested that you concentrate too much on this area, to the exclusion of task — that is, the jobs that actually need to be done.

Your answers to this Activity may well have reflected some of the areas for development that you identified during the goal-setting exercise on management skills that you did as part of your Personal Profile at the start of the programme. If they did not, you may wish to go back to your profile at this stage and review some of your goals and action plans.

HOW MUCH SHOULD YOU CHANGE?

One question which arises from Activity 5 is how far it is possible to change behaviour — something which may be deeply rooted in your background and personality. You may have felt that your style is actually the most effective for some situations, and that it would be a mistake to try to change it.

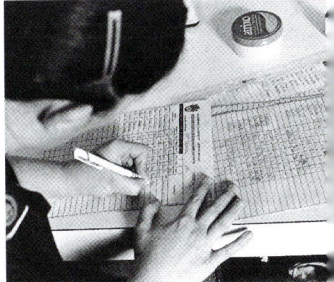

We want to explore the idea that a good manager behaves differently in different circumstances, choosing the style that is most appropriate to each different situation he/she faces. By doing this, we hope to show that you may be able to adapt your management behaviour in some situations.

The things which managers have to deal with arise out of a combination of three factors:

- The tasks to be done

- The people who have to do them

- The managers themselves.

As we have seen, most management decisions are about choosing the best way to juggle these three factors in a way which is beneficial to the organisation (the quality aspects), and acceptable to all concerned.

In the late fifties, Tannenbaum and Schmidt[4] developed a scale of styles reflecting the range of different approaches to decision-making. This scale is shown in the diagram below:

Fig. 2. Management styles

Use of authority by manager						
						Area of freedom for subordinates
1	2	3	4	5	6	7
Manager makes decision, tells group	Manager 'sells' decision to group	Manager makes decision, invites comment	Manager presents problem, gets ideas, makes decisions	Manager joins group, group decides	Manager defines limits, group decides	Manager allows defined area of freedom

The styles to the left of the diagram, in which the manager is a stronger influence than the needs of the people working for him or her, are called *autocratic*. As we move to the right of the diagram, other members of the manager's team get progressively more say in decisions, and the manager's style becomes more *democratic*.

Very few managers will use one style to the exclusion of all the others, although as we saw in Activity 4 above, most will feel more comfortable operating within a narrow range. Your position on the matrix in Figure 1 may help you to decide which styles in Figure 2 you are most likely to use.

ACTIVITY 6
diary
Look at Figure 2 and make a note of the description on the scale which you think best fits your management 'style'.

FEEDBACK

If you showed a high concern for 'task' in Activity 4, you probably identified a style towards the left, or 'autocratic', end of Figure 2. If you showed a high concern for 'people' in Activity 4 you are more likely to have identified a style towards the right, or 'democratic' end of the scale.

In recent years many professionals have written about different learning styles. The American professor David Kolb has been particularly influential in this area and you might like to read his book on experiential learning[5].

Now would be a good moment to take a look at your time log analysis from *M1(i): Are you a manager?* and to place some of the concepts you have been looking at in your actual work situation.

If you have had time to complete the Focus Activity in *M1(i): Are you a manager?* you will have discovered what happens to your time and you will also be able to see those areas where there is a delicate balance between dealing with people and dealing with tasks or activities.

ACTIVITY 7
diary
Make a list of any examples of 'people management' issues of this nature which emerged from your time log analysis. If you have not yet managed to complete the time log, try the Activity anyway, using your past experience as a source of ideas.

Reaching a Decision

ACTIVITY 8
discussion
Go back to your list from Activity 7. For each of the people management issues you wrote down, look again at the 'Comments/Outcomes' column of your time log analysis (or use your past experience to identify typical outcomes). Then make a note of which quarter of the matrix in Figure 1 reflects the way you handled the situation. You may find it useful to discuss these situations with your practice supervisor or other mentor.

We suggested earlier that a good manager will adopt the style which is most appropriate to a given situation, and that the nature of each situation is determined by the interplay between three forces:

- The manager's style

- The capabilities and expectations of the other members of their team

- The nature of the job to be done.

ACTIVITY 9
diary
Look back to the holiday rota problem you considered in Activity 2.
Make brief notes on the nature of the job. Then assess the capabilities and expectations of the other members of the team. Finally, select the management style on the scale in Figure 2 which you think would be the best one to deal with this particular situation.

FEEDBACK

The 'nature of the job to be done' includes both the production of a holiday rota which all the members of the team accept and are happy with, and the maintenance of staffing levels which will enable the organisation to function effectively throughout the holiday period. There is no immediate urgency to complete the rota, but it will have to be completed within a specific time-span (that is, before the holiday period starts).

In this particular scenario, the other members of the team would certainly expect to be consulted about the holiday rota, and would probably be able to come up with their own suggestions about how the problem could be dealt with.

Looking at Figure 2, styles 4, 5 and 6 might all be appropriate in this situation, but you may have concluded that, as a manager, styles 4 and 5 might take up more of your time than you could spare, and that you might get into the difficult position of having to decide between the claims of one member of your team and another. Style 6, where the members of the group are told clearly about the minimum staffing requirements, and then reach a decision themselves, is probably the best approach here.

So we can see that by analysing each management decision, and adopting the style which is appropriate to it, we may be able to change our management behaviour some of the time, while retaining the parts of it which we feel work pretty well for us the rest of the time.

As you have worked through the Activities on management style, you may well have felt that in your particular organisation, people don't get much opportunity to develop an individual management style, and that there are factors within the organisation which control the way people who work for it manage.

MANAGING AND THE ORGANISATION

In the 1960s, management researchers[6, 7] suggested that the way managers manage is largely determined by the sort of organisation they work for, and that some organisations make it easier for individual managers to manage than others. Let's explore this further by thinking about the word 'easy'.

FEEDBACK

ACTIVITY 10
diary
What factors do you think would make it 'easy' for a manager to manage? What might make it less 'easy'.

Although most managers would probably deny that management is ever easy, we can identify some aspects of the job which could make life simpler for an individual manager.

You might have suggested that being clear about what has to be done, and exactly how much responsibility the manager is expected to shoulder, are important factors in making a manager's life 'easier'. You might also have suggested that having a certain amount of freedom to exercise individual style would also be important.

Task Structure

Some writers on management[7] have suggested that it is easier to manage when the jobs to be done, and who is responsible for them, are clearly spelt out and understood by all concerned.

This spelling out of the jobs to be done has been called the *task structure* of the organisation. Some types of work are better suited to having a clearly defined task structure than others.

EXAMPLES

The flight crews of passenger aeroplanes will have strict procedures to cover all phases of the flight: checks and counter-checks, emergency procedures and so on, to make sure that every step is taken to ensure the safety of passengers.

On the other hand, a team of writers and artists working on an advertising campaign might have a much looser structure of tasks and responsibilities, allowing much more scope for individual creativity or group work.

ACTIVITY 11
diary
Think about the task structure in your own area of work. Are individual tasks clearly spelt out? Is each task the responsibility of a specific person or group? Make some notes in your diary about whether you think this is the most appropriate task structure for the work which has to be done.

FEEDBACK

Your thoughts on this will depend very much on the type of healthcare environment in which you work. Nursing in an acute area may demand a much more clearly defined task structure than nursing in residential care, for example.

Healthcare organisations as a whole tend to have fairly rigid task structures and, depending on where you work, you may have reflected that the task structure of your organisation is too rigid for the type of care you provide, making the work of managing more difficult. On the other hand, you may have concluded that the type of work in which you are involved requires a fairly clear definition of tasks and responsibilities.

Position Power

Organisations which have a relatively rigid task structure often also have clearly identified ranks and disciplinary codes. Such organisations will also be more likely to use the wearing of uniforms as a means of reinforcing this structure. Fiedler[8] also gives a label to these means of reinforcing the task structure. He calls it position power, and he maintains that a strong position power in an organisation makes the job of managers easier.

ACTIVITY 12
diary
What indications of position power are used in your organisation? Do you consider that they make life easier or more difficult for those (including you) who manage at any level in the organisation?

FEEDBACK

Once again, your answers will depend on the type of organisation you work for. Traditionally, healthcare organisations tend to be strong on factors such as rank, and the wearing of uniforms. However, it is becoming more common for certain types of healthcare organisations to abandon some of the trappings of position power; for example, the wearing of uniforms in homes for the care of terminally ill patients.

As in our discussion of management styles above, we can see that no one type of organisational structure is necessarily 'better' or 'worse' to manage than others. What is important is that the structure is appropriate for what the organisation is trying to do.

ACTIVITY 13
diary
If you have worked in more than one healthcare organisation (including those you experienced during your training), write down how it felt to work in each of them. If the atmosphere differed, make a note of what you think caused this. Did each organisation have a distinctive management style and, if so, can you describe it?

We will be exploring some more detailed questions about the most appropriate way to manage the care we provide in other Parts of the Management module.

We end this Part by considering the most important factor in any manager's life — the people he or she has to work with. This will lead in to *M2: Teamwork.*

THE PEOPLE FACTOR

In most fields of human activity, the behaviour of people is the variable which is most difficult to predict and control. Because of this, managers in organisations may find it difficult to judge how employees will react to change, such as the introduction of new technology or work procedures.

ACTIVITY 14
diary
Can you think of any examples from your own workplace where people reacted to change:
(a) well?
(b) badly?
Can you suggest why each of these reactions occurred?

FEEDBACK

You may have found it easy to identify examples in Activity 14, but less easy to pin down reasons for different reactions to change.

Response to change, and the reaction of management to that response, is more likely to be favourable if an organisation has what Fiedler[8] has called good leader-member relations. This means how well the manager gets on with the rest of the team, and what they think of the manager. Despite the importance of the other organisational factors we have considered this week, interpersonal relationships are really the key to successful management.

Notes

ACTIVITY 15
discussion

Look back to your answers to Activities 7 and 8. Make notes on how you intend in the future to approach the interpersonal management issues you raised. You may want to think again about the management style you used for each issue in your list from Activity 7.

Are there any other factors in the organisation you work for which might influence your approach?

To help consolidate all you have covered in this Part, talk to your practice supervisor about the way you intend to approach these management issues in the future.

The Focus asks you to identify some of the management issues in your own workplace which will be central to your work in the rest of the Management module.

Many trusts have applied for the Investors in People (IIP) benchmark. IIP recognises that people are the best asset any organisation has and provides a framework for creating a people-centred organisation. You might like to find out more about IIP and check out whether your organisation has achieved the IIP award or has embarked on the IIP process.

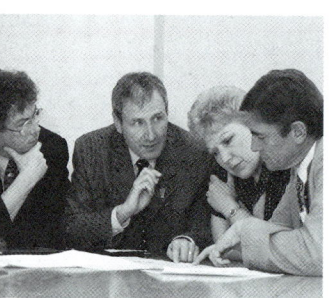

FOCUS

Look back through this Part and *M1(i): Are you a manager?* on principles of management. We have raised a number of important issues about:

- The nature of your job

- Your own personality and style of management.

Reflect on your own work situation and identify any management issues which you think could be resolved to improve the standard of healthcare you provide. There might be issues relating to how you manage your own work, or to how the team in which you work is managed.

Make some notes about these, detailing what the problem is, what you consider the management issues to be, and what questions you need answers to in order to resolve the problem.

We will be referring to these issues throughout the Management module.

REFERENCES

1 Fleishman, E.A., Harris, E.F. Patterns of leadership behaviour related to employee grievance and turnover. *Personnel Psychology* 1962; 15: 43–56.

2 Mouton, J.S., Blake, R.R. *The Managerial Grid III.* Houston: Gulf Publishing, 1984; page 10.

3 Reddin, W.J. *Managerial Effectiveness.* New York: McGraw-Hill, 1970.

4 Tannenbaum, R., Schmidt, W.H. How to choose a leadership pattern. *Harvard Business Review* 1958; **36**: 2, 95–101.

5 Kolb, D. *Experiential Learning: Experience as the source of learning and development.* New Jersey: Pentrice Hall, 1986.

6 Woodward, J. *Industrial Organisation: Behaviour and control.* Oxford: Oxford University Press, 1970.

7 Burns, T., Stalker, G.M. *The Management of Innovation.* London: Tavistock, 1961.

8 Fiedler, F.E., Chemers, M.M. *Leadership and Effective Management.* New York: Scott Foresman & Co, 1974.

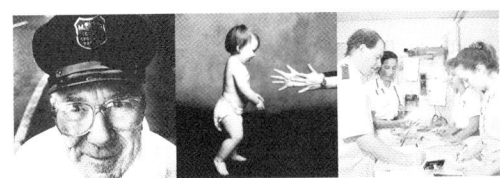

Term 3

The third term brings into focus particular aspects of the level-1 nurse. We start by exploring issues relating to client assessment (P5), building on the ideas about individual attitudes to health and healthcare that we discussed in Term 1.

Section P6 looks at how we can help others to learn — an important aspect of the level-1 nurse. These ideas are developed further in P7 when we explore some of the issues surrounding your role in health promotion and how to plan and implement such a programme.

We end by helping you to become familiar with different research approaches you might encounter in your practice. You will explore different views which researchers can have of their subject matter, and examine how their choice of approach can influence the methods they use to carry out research.

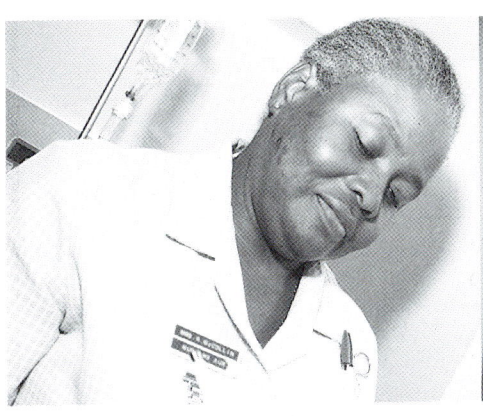
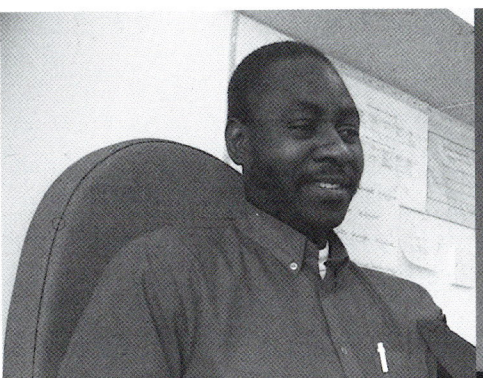
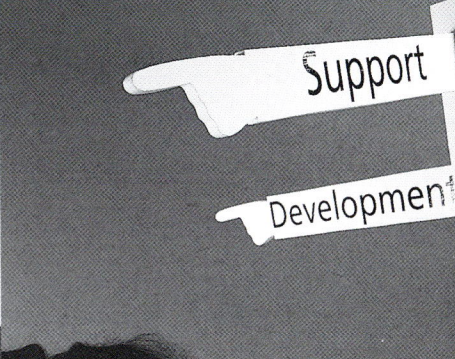

Assessment in context

You make assessments in your everyday life all the time. As a nurse, you assess your clients and their needs as part of the process of providing care.

In this Part you will think about:

- The process of making assessments in everyday and nursing life
- How your opinions of other people, and their view of you, can colour the information you give and receive
- The consequences of making a wrong assessment
- Making assessments in nursing.

WORK PLANNER

Before starting work on this Part, look at the ideas we explored in *P2: Human Biography*. They provide a foundation for the work here.

In Activity 2 you are asked to involve a friend or family member in making an assessment of you. You may want to make arrangements in advance.

In Activity 5 and the Focus you are asked to discuss some of the issues raised with your tutor/counsellor. You should arrange to meet him or her, or make contact by telephone, while you are working on this Part.

THE PROCESS OF ASSESSMENT

We make assessments all the time in our everyday lives as well as at work. We 'assess' whether the carrots in the supermarket are a better buy than those in the greengrocer, whether we have time to go to the post office on the way home from work, and so on. Most of these assessments are made subconsciously.

Everyday decisions such as these are usually based on our own assessment of a situation. They do not directly involve asking someone else's opinion to help us decide. When we make an assessment like this, we draw upon our existing knowledge base and gather any new knowledge or information we need to help us make sense of the situation and decide what choices are open to us.

EXAMPLE

If you are deciding whether to buy South African Granny Smith apples or English Cox's, you might consider the following in making your assessment of the alternatives:

What you already know about apples

- The kind of apple you know you like — sweet, crisp, one which will last a few days without turning into cotton wool

- Your experience of both of these types of apple.

Additional information you need to make the assessment

- How many apples you need

- How much money you have to spend

- How many you will get to the pound

- What these particular apples look like — do they look fresh and appetising, or tired and dry?

- Perhaps it is necessary to buy one of each and try them first.

Your own values, attitudes and beliefs

- You may believe that British is best and that British products should be supported wherever possible.

This type of everyday assessment is pretty straightforward; however, there are other assessments we make, often more important ones, which involve gathering information from other people, who may or may not be affected by the decisions we make.

EXAMPLES

Assessments like this may include where we should live, whether we should make a job change, which school we should send our five-year-old to, which doctor we should register with, even what to do about a relationship that seems to be going wrong.

ACTIVITY 1
diary

Think of two decisions you have made in which the assessment process involved seeking information from other people:
(a) One where the people who gave you information were not affected by your decision
(b) One where the people who gave you information were affected by your final decision.
In both cases describe the various factors you took into account when gathering the information and assessing the pros and cons.

The process of making these kinds of assessments and the decisions based on them is exactly the same as we described with the apples: a course of action is needed; we draw upon our existing knowledge base in relation to the situation; we gather information from a variety of sources, one of which is the opinion of other people.

Using people as sources of information introduces another element into the assessment process: how they see us and assess what they think we want to know. What they tell us will also be influenced by whether or not they will be personally affected by any decision we make. How we are feeling when we make the decision becomes more important here — if we are stressed, in a hurry or distracted, this could influence our own interpretation of that information.

HOW OTHERS SEE US

In *P2: Human Biography*, we looked at the way we see situations and other people and at how our views are coloured as a result of our life experience.

ACTIVITY 2
action
Write down how you see a particular aspect of yourself. It may be your looks, health, level of fitness, levels of tolerance, your taste in clothes, or your career potential.
Now ask a friend or a member of your family to describe how they see this particular aspect of you.
Did you find any variations between your assessment and theirs?
Can you suggest any reason for this?

CASE STUDY

Louise and **Jane** have been friends and colleagues for some time, working closely on a major project. However, they have never visited each other's homes, or met each other's families. The two women are the same age and Jane assessed that, on the whole, they would probably have similar ideas on issues relating to family and life-style. Jane sees Louise as a working mother with a grown-up family, practical and down-to-earth like herself. However, Jane's assessment was shaken when Louise turned up one day in a two-seater sports car, and explained to a stunned Jane that the second family car was also a soft-top sports saloon. Not a very big issue perhaps, but Jane did not see Louise as a sports car enthusiast!

Louise was surprised to find that Jane had always seen her as what Louise herself would have described as a 'boring, middle-class housewife'. Other people's opinions of us matter a great deal to us personally, especially those whom we consider close friends, family or colleagues.

We all have the tendency to label people according to the way they look, speak and act, and adapt our advice and service accordingly. Unfortunately, this can sometimes be costly in time and money and can create disharmony and unhappiness.

A nurse lecturer has described in an article how he used a local theatre group to help student nurses gain valuable perspectives on community health issues[1].

WHAT IS THE REAL SITUATION?

As explained in *P2: Human Biography*, we all see life, people and situations differently as a result of our life experience, and the mutual knowledge of our social group. Therefore it could be argued that our idea of 'reality' could, in certain situations, be open to challenge[2].

People often try to make sense of situations by drawing on their past experience. Some social scientists[2] believe that we give our own meaning to people, things and actions and that in so doing we create our own 'reality', which, in certain situations, could be open to challenge by others[3].

Notes

Many people adopt roles in response to a new or difficult situation which are very different from their normal behaviour.

EXAMPLES

The dynamic businesswoman who behaves like a submissive female with men in a social situation; the man who cannot manage when asked to run the home for a day; the person who copes with situations in which his or her independence is threatened by becoming withdrawn and aggressive. At the start of the Open Learning programme you may have adopted the role of 'student', based on your expectations about what being a student means.

Other people react to what they see as being reality and assess the situation and the person accordingly.

EXAMPLE

The man meeting the businesswoman for the first time responds to the reality she has created, and treats her as a 'submissive female'; the community midwife, seeing the helpless male running the home single-handed, bustles around him offering help and advice; the nurse reacts angrily to the aggressive person, not seeing the underlying anxiety.

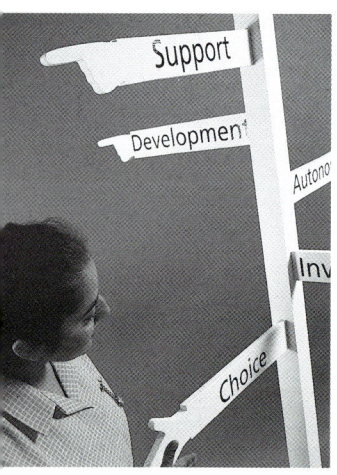

ASSESSMENT IN NURSING

We have seen so far that we use the process of assessment all the time in our everyday lives, and we have explored some of the factors which can affect the nature of the assessments we make. We have seen, in particular, that information from other people, whether they are affected by our final decision or not, can often be influenced by their perceptions of us and what they think we want to know. The information they supply based on these assumptions may have a marked effect on the decision we end up making.

These factors play a particularly important part in the assessments we make as nurses.

Most of us use a systematic, problem-solving approach when we make decisions in our personal and professional lives. In other words, we assess a situation, devise a plan of action, implement it and evaluate it. This may happen with any of our dealings with other staff, clients' families and friends, when helping students develop skills, and in providing a service for our clients.

Using information based on inaccurate information can be a waste of valuable time and resources, and, if the wrong type of care is chosen as a result, can also include added suffering for the client and his or her family.

P5(ii): Client assessment in practice looks more closely at assessment in nursing.

If you are interested in learning more about assessment of your own learning, and about some of the different types of assessment we can use for this, look at *Assessment and Learning*[4], one of Emap Healthcare Open Learning's Professional Practice Study Units.

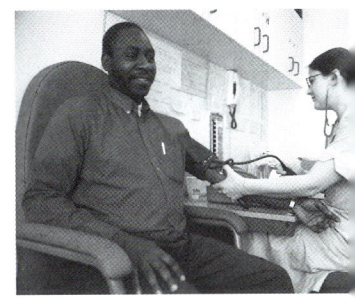

FOCUS

Think of three decisions you have made at work in the past week. Make some notes in your diary about the process you went through in each case: how much background information you had on which to base your assessment and decision; how you went about seeking any additional information, and from what source; whether your own, or other people's, values attitudes and beliefs played a part; the sort of environment in which you made each decision (that is, were you stressed, did you have plenty of time to consider the information you had, and so on?). How confident are you that the decision you made was the right one in each case?

Discuss your evaluation of these three decisions with your tutor/counsellor.

REFERENCES

1   Hurst, B. Drama class. *Nursing Times* 1993; **89**: 1, 30–31.

2   Thomas, N.I. *The Unadjusted Girl*. New York: Harper & Row, 1967.

3   Aggleton, P., Chalmers, H. *Nursing Models and the Nursing Process*. London: Macmillan Education Ltd, 1986.

4   Macmillan Open Learning [Emap Healthcare Open Learning]. *Assessment and Learning*. Professional practice study unit: Teaching and Learning in Practice. London: Macmillan Magazines Ltd., 1996.

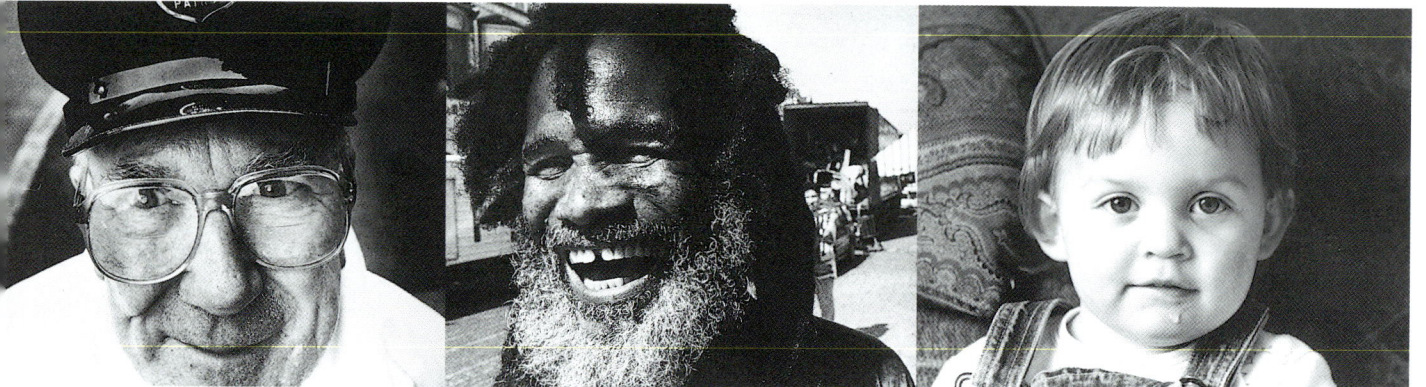

Notes

Client assessment in practice

In this second Part of *P5: Client Assessment*, you will see that the way you assess clients in relation to their experiences and expectations can affect client care and well-being.

You will look at a number of key aspects of client assessment:

- Generalising versus individual needs
- The client's own experiences and expectations
- Getting the right information about the client's situation
- Passing on information
- Evaluating your assessments.

WORK PLANNER

Activity 3 asks you to identify two people in different age groups who are or have been in hospital, and to ask them how they feel about the health care they received. We suggest that you avoid using any clients who are under your own personal care at present. If possible, use friends, relatives or colleagues for this Activity.

The Focus asks you to discuss a particular client or situation with a colleague. Before you do this, make sure that the person you choose is clear about the importance of maintaining confidentiality on the subject.

Whatever your position and level of responsibility, you are required to make assessments every day in your nursing practice. You make decisions about a whole range of things at work: patient care, prioritising your work, whose advice and guidance to seek, how best to help a student nurse develop a new skill, and so on, based on the information which you already have, or are able to collect about the situation.

Most of what we say here relates to the way we assess the healthcare needs of our patients or clients, but as you work through it you should bear in mind that it can relate just as much to decisions about your own work, or about colleagues.

ASSESSING CLIENTS AND THEIR NEEDS

In our work as nurses, we often have very little time, and very little background knowledge of patients or clients, when making our initial assessments, and we often find ourselves relying on previous experiences to make sense of what is going on in the present. One of the ways we do this is to *generalise*.

Making generalisations about other people is almost an automatic process. With limited information about our clients, at least when we first meet them, our initial assessment is often based on our subconscious ideas and experience of other people we consider to be similar.

Most of us work in settings where some members of our client group have some things in common, and we therefore generalise about certain aspects of their care.

CASE STUDY

Christine was a midwife who was booked to have her baby in the unit where she had worked before she married. This was her third uneventful pregnancy. Her two previous births had been easy and uncomplicated. In the event, this one also went smoothly — so smoothly, in fact, that none of the midwives on duty realised that her labour was progressing rapidly. Seeing her calmly walking about, or knitting, the midwives assumed that she was still in the early stages of labour. They were therefore surprised when, during the registrar's round, Christine sat down and announced that she was ready to push the baby out.

The midwives later admitted that because Christine was an ex-midwife, and from the unit, they were convinced that they were going to 'have trouble with her'. 'She's a midwife, so things are bound to go wrong' was the general view, based on a sort of myth which had grown up in the unit, part of the mutual knowledge of that group of midwives, that the more you knew about childbirth, the more likely things were to go wrong.

ACTIVITY 1
diary
Think of some of the generalisations that are made about your particular client group. Write two of them down, and note whether you can honestly say that you have ever had cause to doubt them.

Generalising about the care needs of groups of people can mean that their individual needs are overlooked.

CASE STUDY

Mary was 77, fit and agile until the day she tripped and fell while running to catch a bus, and fractured her neck of femur. She spent three days in hospital in pain and confusion, waiting for an operation. Her daughter, a nurse, visited her each day. When Mary finally received her operation, the surgeons inserted a partial hip replacement, on the grounds that, because of her age, she would lead a fairly inactive life-style. Six months after surgery, Mary was still using sticks, and was in considerable pain. She caught her foot on uneven flooring at her local supermarket, and fell again, this time injuring her back. She was disappointed and anxious about her poor recovery, and saw her consultant again. Her daughter asked whether the treatment she had received was the most appropriate for her life-style. The consultant told them that as Mary was over 75, it was assumed she would not be doing much walking, or would be in a home, and treated accordingly. He also told her to stop blaming the original accident for her falls. 'You are old, and when you get old, you fall over a lot.' Mary had never fallen in her life before. She has now lost her self-esteem and self-confidence. At 80 years of age, she is still waiting her turn for a full hip replacement to ease her pain and, in her words: 'to get back to where I was before my accident', three years ago.

Notes

Mary was the victim of a policy which generalised about people over a certain age, and which clearly took no account of the individual. Despite the fact that Mary waited three days for surgery, no one asked Mary or her daughter what her usual life-style and activity was like.

ACTIVITY 2
diary
Can you think of any similar incidents, either
(a) where you or a member of your family was a client, or
(b) involving one of your clients where generalising about the needs of a group led to inappropriate individual needs being identified? Make some notes in your diary.

Some of the situations you manage as a nurse require you to make, and act upon, assessments quickly: for example, when a patient is admitted haemorrhaging, or a patient has a cardiac arrest in the ward bathroom. In situations like these you have to act quickly: assess the situation, decide what has to be done, who should do it, and then get on with it.

However, in most other cases, you have more time to gather information about the individual, and in particular the kind of biographical information which would give you a better understanding of how the client sees nurses, what is happening, and what he or she expects will happen.

THE CLIENT'S VIEWPOINT

It is important to remember that just as we, as nurses, often make judgements about groups, or types of patients, using generalisations based on our past experience, so our clients, too, are assessing us and the situation in which they find themselves.

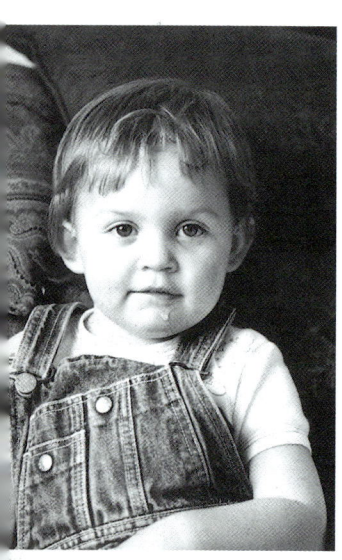

ACTIVITY 3
action
Think of two people you know, preferably in different age groups, who are, or have been, patients in hospital. Write down in your diary how you think they feel/felt about needing treatment; how they feel about hospitals; how they see doctors and nurses: what they believe each of these groups does and is responsible for; what they expect the health service to provide for them. When you have completed your notes, ask the people themselves to tell you how they feel about all these elements, and compare their answers with your notes.

FEEDBACK

You may have found that there were many areas in which your opinions and feelings were broadly similar. However, this Activity may also have highlighted how each of us can see the same situation differently, and in particular how different people's views and expectations affect the way they view their health care.

Different People, Different Expectations

Faced with the prospect of a stay in hospital — an alien environment to many — people will often try to make sense of it through their personal history and experience. For example, a patient may adopt a submissive role, transferring the roles of her parents when she was a child to the doctors and nurses, expecting to do as she is told, and putting her welfare in the hands of her 'parents'. On the other hand, previous experience may dictate that she behaves in entirely the opposite way:

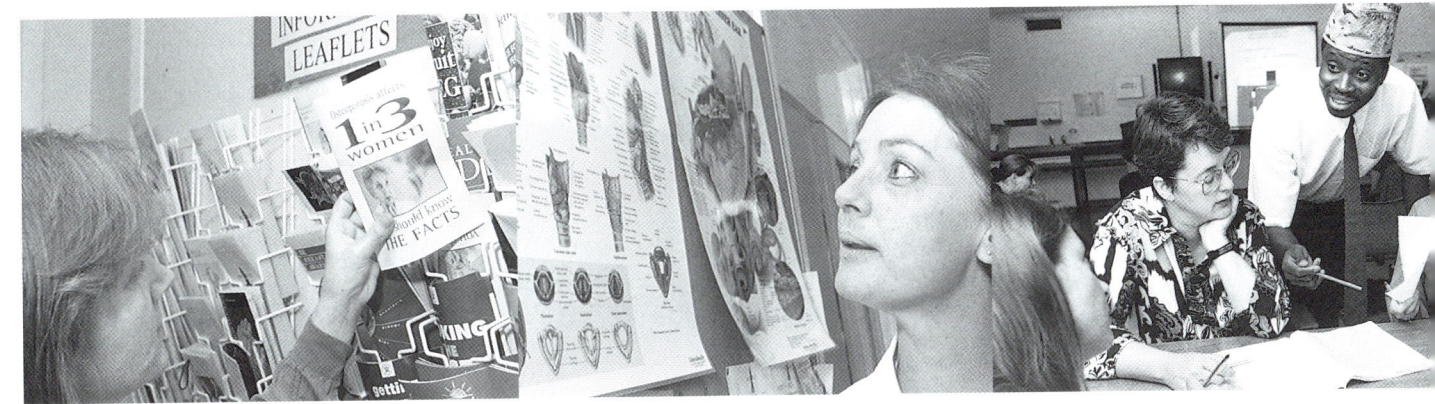

Learning and communication

Part of the role of the qualified clinical nurse is teaching students. But, as nurses, there are other groups with whom we come into contact and whom we can also help to learn — our colleagues and clients. Here and in *P6(ii): The process of facilitation* we explore the role of the nurse as being someone who can help others to learn, and find out how we can improve our own communication skills to make us better able to do this.

You will consider:

- How people learn
- The groups of people you help to learn and how you do this
- The key skills of a facilitator
    - listening and attending
    - using questions.

WORK PLANNER

Before you start work on this Part, take some time to look back over:

- Section 4 of the Review in the Profile Pack: 'What kind of learner are you?'
- The Foundation Section of this book: *Responding to Change*.

The Focus Activity asks you to choose two people — a colleague and a client — to talk about their learning needs. You may want to identify these people and schedule some time with them in advance.

You may also want to refresh your memory on some points made about open learning in Moya Davis's book, *A Student's Guide to Open Learning*, which is part of this conversion programme's support material.

You may also find it useful to read a handbook on communication skills. *People Skills* by Robert Bolton, published by Simon and Schuster Inc., (1986) is a practical book which you can read right through or dip into.

HOW DO PEOPLE LEARN?

Facilitating learning means helping other people to learn. In following this programme of open learning, you are being helped to learn in a particular way: studying at your own pace, and being able to choose when and where you study.

Giving learners more control over their own learning, as we have done with this programme, is one way of creating an *environment* which encourages learning. Here the

149

focus is on how you can help people learn, and how you can create environments in which they can learn more easily.

Throughout our lives, we learn an enormous amount. Some things we are taught, others we learn from other people, or from our own experience. Some things we learn through *formal* methods, such as those at school, or on training courses; others we learn through *informal* methods, such as discussing things with friends and colleagues, watching television, or by actually doing things for ourselves.

ACTIVITY 1
diary
Choose two learning experiences which were successful for you. These may be ones you have already thought about in other units, or in your Profile, or you may wish to select new ones. Try to choose one where you learnt something *formally,* and one where you learnt *informally.* Think about how you learnt these things. Identify factors in the learning environment (the people, the resources, the place) and factors in you (your motivation, your goals) which contributed to your learning.

FEEDBACK

Learning is a product of the two elements we have identified in this Activity — the learning environment and the learner. An effective facilitator of learning is one who combines these two to best effect. We can't know what you put in answer to the above Activity — it could have been anything from spending time with your favourite uncle as a child, so learning from his tales of his youth, to looking forward to lessons with the only teacher in the school who talked to you as a person rather than handing out endless worksheets and leaving you to get on with it.

A good facilitator understands learners' goals (what they want to learn) and their motivation (why they want to learn), and finds the best way of enabling them to achieve those goals. Some of the people who helped you to learn in the past may have done so unconsciously, not realising that they had said or done something which made things 'click' for you. Or the learning may have arisen almost by accident — your interest in a subject was aroused, and the facilitator was able to help in exactly the right way.

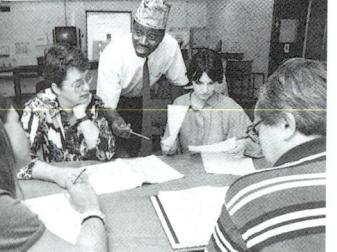

WHO ARE YOUR LEARNERS?

We know that as a first-level nurse your job will involve helping students to learn. This is an important part of your role, and one for which you will probably receive more training after you have qualified. But we would also like to suggest that in the course of your practice many other groups will be able to learn from you.

ACTIVITY 2
diary
Which other people do you think could learn from you at work?

The Research module explores the existence of a body of specialised 'nursing' knowledge. Some of this knowledge consists of facts and skills that you know to be true, either from what you have been taught or have learnt from your own experience in nursing practice. Other nursing knowledge consists of mutual nursing knowledge — the attitudes which you hold in common with other nurses about the 'best' way of doing things, or about your relationships with other healthcare professionals, your clients and patients, the general public, and so on.

In possession of this specialised knowledge — these 'nursing' facts, skills and attitudes — you might be in a position to help a number of other groups of people to learn. These might include, for example, professional colleagues (doctors, nurses, social workers, and so on), auxiliary staff, clients and their families.

ACTIVITY 3
diary
Make some notes about how each of the following groups is helped to learn, either by you or others, in your current practice.
• Students • Other professional colleagues • Auxiliary staff • Clients and their families.

FEEDBACK

On the whole, students still learn mainly by formal methods — watching other nurses in practice, attending demonstrations, lectures, seminars, and so on. However, as you will have discovered in your work on the programme, there are many ways in which learning can be more student-centred, with learners having more say about when and what they learn. This means that people other than those responsible for the students' formal learning may also have a role to play as facilitators, and this could include you.

Informal learning is much more likely to occur in the case of your colleagues or auxiliary staff. As we have said above, nursing knowledge has much to offer other professionals, and even as qualified nurses we can always learn more from each other if we can identify opportunities to do so.

In the case of clients, you may have said that you already do a fair amount to help them to learn.

ACTIVITY 4
diary
What do you consider to be the main purpose of helping clients to learn more about their condition or treatment? Describe the methods currently used in your workplace to facilitate learning in your clients and their families.

FEEDBACK

Helping clients and their families to understand more about their condition or treatment will help them take more control over their own care. This understanding can be increased simply by providing *information*, either formally or informally, and much of the health education that nurses are involved in comes into this category. However, we can also influence our clients' attitudes to themselves and their care by informal methods. *P6(ii): The process of facilitation* explores ways in which we can recognise and use opportunities to help others to learn.

FACILITATION SKILLS

Facilitation is about helping people to discover things for themselves rather than telling them things. *P1(ii): Health and power* considers the nurse's position as an expert, and discusses the dangers of using that position to force our opinions and attitudes on others by simply telling them what to do and expecting them to accept it because we speak from a position of authority.

ACTIVITY 5
diary
Reflect for a few minutes on two teachers you have known — one whom you consider to have been a 'good' teacher and one whom you consider to have been a 'bad' teacher. What were their teaching styles? Did they tell you things, or did they encourage you to puzzle things out for yourself?

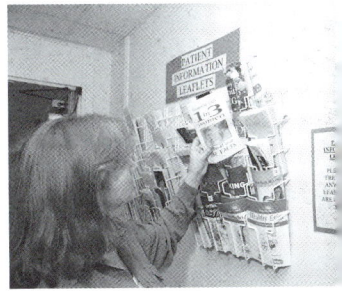

A 'good' teacher for one person may not necessarily be a 'good' teacher for someone else. We all have our own individual learning needs. For example, some people are comfortable learning facts and then being encouraged to analyse, while others prefer to work things out for themselves. Some people learn well by open learning, while others prefer closer contact with other students and tutors.

Becoming a facilitator involves adopting a certain frame of mind. It involves finding out the learners' motivation — what it is that will make them want to learn — and then deciding on the best way of helping them. This may involve standing back and encouraging them to inquire about what they are seeing and doing, or it may involve providing information and feedback on something specific.

Two key skills of a good facilitator are:

- Listening and attending

- Using questions.

You will now look at these two skills and think about:

- How much you use them yourself at present

- How much more you could use them in the future.

Listening and Attending

To listen actively to another person is one of the most caring acts of all. We show that we are interested in that person as another human being. It is not sufficient just to sit and look at the other person and to nod occasionally. We must give him/her our full attention.

Many things may get in the way of this process, and prevent us from listening even if we are trying hard to pay attention. A short list of such things would be:

- Lack of time

- External distractions, such as background noise or movement

- Our personal feelings either for or against the person who is talking

- Our own feelings and emotions about the subject being discussed

- Our personal feelings about the situation (for example, we might feel that we are not the most appropriate person to deal with what is being talked about)

- Rehearsing what we are going to say when the other person stops talking

- Anything else going on in our heads at the same time.

The person to whom we are listening may also put up blocks, either consciously or unconsciously, and obscure the meaning of what he has to say. The person may:

- Have language problems, and be unable to make himself understood

- Have feelings about us, and our status as nurses, which prevent him from stating his views and feelings clearly

- Be so immersed in the issue that he is unable to state his needs clearly.

Overcoming the barriers to listening which we have listed above takes patience and practice. Some of the work in other units will contribute to this: *P2: Human Biography* and *P5: Client Assessment* explored how all people's feelings are shaped by their backgrounds and their attitudes to different social groups.

Good listening skills

ACTIVITY 6
diary
Think about two of your friends and two of your colleagues. Which of them (if any) would you nominate as 'good listeners'? What characteristics did you use to make your choice?

FEEDBACK

People who are thought of as good listeners usually manage to convey a feeling of being relaxed, of having enough time to give to the other person. They do this by outward signs such as smiles and nods, by not interrupting, and by conveying appropriate responses to what the other person is saying.

A number of ways of showing you are listening involve using appropriate body language, using your body to give non-verbal signals that you are listening. Egan[1] suggests that the following behaviours convey to a person that he is being listened to:

S Sitting *squarely* in relation to the other person. Sit across from, rather than next to him. In this way, both of you see each other clearly.

O Maintaining an '*open*' position: crossed arms and legs may signify defensiveness on the part of the listener.

L *Leaning* slightly towards the person who is talking. This helps to reinforce the fact that you are interested in both the person and in listening to him.

E Maintaining comfortable *eye contact*. To listen to another person involves looking at him. However, don't stare or maintain a fixed gaze; merely be ready to meet his eyes as they look at you.

R *Relaxing.* People never feel they are being listened to if they feel hurried. If you are really going to listen to the person in front of you, allow yourself to take a couple of deep breaths and enjoy the time that you spend with each other.

This is just one 'system' which you could adopt: you may not be comfortable with some of the suggestions in Egan's list, but the whole point is to let the other person know that you are relaxed and interested in what he is saying, and that you have understood what has been said.

ACTIVITY 7
discussion
How good a listener are you? Make notes about the things that make it difficult for you to listen. Also note down what you consider to be your strengths as a listener. Then ask a good friend what she thinks of you as a listener. Does your friend see you as an effective listener?

There are a number of ways in which you can develop and practise listening skills, apart from rehearsing your body language. Radio and television can be used to good effect, and Activity 8 gives some suggestions.

ACTIVITY 8
action
The following are suggestions as to how you can practise your listening skills.
1. Listen to a short talk on the radio, and record it at the same time. When it has finished, make notes about the main points covered, then play back your recording to check how well you listened to what was said.
2. Watch people talking on television, but with the sound turned down. Try to work out the tone of the conversation from the body language they use. If you videotape it at the same time, you will be able to play it back later to check how well you read the non-verbal signals used.

Listening is an important skill in facilitating learning, because it allows the other person to think through his concerns, ideas and feelings, and allows you to discover the learner's needs and motivation.

Using Questions

The use of questions is also important to the listening process for the facilitator, and we will look at this skill next. An appropriately phrased question can help others to expand their ideas, develop new theories and become critical of what they are doing.

There are three types of question:

- Open and closed questions

- Reflective questions

- Summarising and checking for understanding.

We will look at each in turn.

Open and closed questions

Closed questions elicit a short answer, usually 'yes' or 'no'. For example: 'Have you checked this with the college of nursing?' 'Did you understand what was said?' 'Is this the information you wanted?'

Open questions invite the other person to give more expansive answers, to offer opinions, and to express his or her own ideas. Open questions usually begin with 'how', 'why', 'what' or 'where'; for example: 'Why did you do that?' 'What sort of support would you like from us on this?' 'How can I help you?'

ACTIVITY 9
knowledge base
How do you think that (a) closed and (b) open questions could be useful to you if you were trying to help someone else to learn?

FEEDBACK

In general, open questions are more facilitative than closed ones, because they encourage learners to explore their own thoughts and views, and to expand on points that may already have been made. However, closed questions are also useful to clarify a point, or to check understanding of specific pieces of information.

Reflective questions

Another type of question which can be used to encourage someone to expand his/her thoughts is the reflective question.

By this stage of the programme, you are probably becoming very familiar with the process of reflection: of continually thinking about what you do, how you do it, and whether you can do it better. Reflection is an important tool for learning, and good facilitators of learning will provide their learners with every opportunity to do it.

Reflective questions are used to 'draw out' another person. They are expressed as a sort of 'echo' of what the person has already said, when you feel that encouragement is needed to say more.

EXAMPLES

'I don't seem to be able to get the hang of this at all ...'
'You can't get the hang of it?'
'No, every new article I read seems to contradict the previous one'.

OR:

'I've tried to reduce the amount of fatty food I eat, but I'm finding it rather difficult at the moment.'
'You find it difficult right now?'
'Yes ... well, my wife has started working longer hours — we need the money, you see — so I've been eating more in the staff canteen, and the food there is always rather greasy. I suppose I could make sandwiches instead.'

ACTIVITY 10
action
Practise using reflective questions today. Make a conscious effort to use them next time you are in conversation with a friend or colleague. At first, you may feel a bit self-conscious but, like all skills, it calls for practice.

Reflective questions sound rather artificial when they appear in print, but they can be very effective when used in conversation.

Summarising and checking for understanding

All the above types of questions can be used to summarise what has been discussed, and to check that you have understood what the learner has said. People often talk rather quickly, and can cover a lot of ground without stopping to consider whether they have been understood or not. Checking for understanding is a way of helping the other person to slow down a little, and to consider in more detail what he or she is saying.

Checking learning in this way is also important for the facilitator as a way of monitoring the learning, and for the learner as a means of measuring progress towards goals.

Closed questions can often be used to great effect.

EXAMPLES

'Let me just check what you are saying. You feel uncomfortable at the moment because you don't feel you are learning anything in this ward. On the other hand, you are not sure who you should discuss this with. Is that a fair summary?'

OR:

'You're not sure about the new drugs and their side-effects, and you haven't been able to find a member of staff who will discuss this with you. Is that what you are saying?'

ACTIVITY 11
action
You can start to practise the skill of checking for understanding next time you are genuinely unclear about something that someone has said to you, either with colleagues, clients or friends.

Practising these skills of listening and questioning whenever you can will prepare you for the role of facilitator when the opportunity arises. *P6(ii): The process of facilitation* explores the idea of learning opportunities, and considers ways in which we can recognise and use such opportunities when they arise.

You might be interested to look at the book *The Practitioner as Teacher*[2], which explores the nature of teaching and learning.

FOCUS

Choose two people, one colleague and one client, whom you think you could help to learn something. In choosing a client, you will probably find it best to select someone with whom you are already working to improve his understanding of his condition or its treatment. You will be asked to work with the same two people again in P6(ii), so make sure that they will be available then.

Make a note in your diary about what it is you think these two people need to learn, and what you think will motivate them to learn.

Now use the skills of listening and asking questions which were discussed in this Part to determine from each of these people what they see as their learning needs for a specific area. For example, for a student it may be learning a new skill, or acquiring more knowledge about a particular area. For a client, it might be more information about his condition, or a health education need.

Now note in your diary whether the learners' needs as they expressed them themselves differed from what *you* thought were their learning needs. If they did differ, suggest reasons why your view was not the same as theirs. Think about the work you did in *P5: Client Assessment* as you do this.

REFERENCES

1   Egan, G. *The Skilled Helper* (4th edn). Pacific Grove, California: Brooks/Cole 1990.
2   Hinchliff, S. (ed.), *The Practitioner as Teacher*. Harrow, Middlesex: Scutari Press, 1992.

155

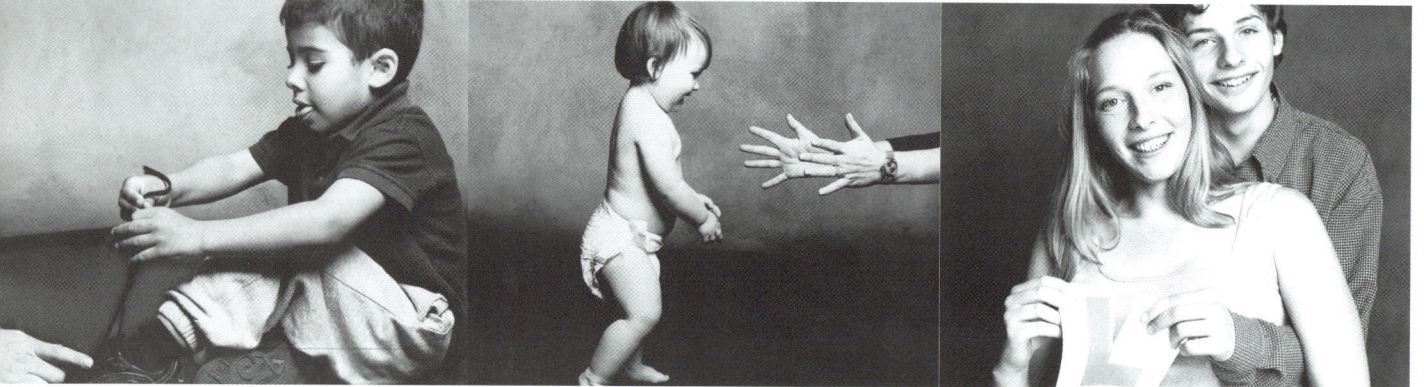

The process of facilitation

As a nurse you have an ongoing role as a learning facilitator. This Part of *P6: Facilitating Learning* considers each stage of the facilitation process. It aims to help you understand what facilitation is, when and how to facilitate learning for other people and how to evaluate your facilitation.

The key stages of the facilitation process are:

- Identifying a learning need
- Setting goals
- Identifying learning resources
- Planning and carrying out the facilitation
- Assessing and evaluating the learning.

WORK PLANNER

In Activity 4 you will return to one of the people whose learning needs you identified in the Focus in *P6(i): Learning and communication*. You will need to schedule one hour with this person to carry out a goal-setting exercise.

In Activity 5 you are asked to explore the learning resources available to you. You will need to plan some time in libraries and resource centres. You might find it helpful to look at the list of resources given in the Activity to give you an idea of what to look for.

P6(i): Learning and communication asked you to think about some of the groups of people whom you could help to learn in the course of your practice as a first-level nurse. It explained that facilitating learning is not just about deciding what needs to be taught and delivering information, but that it is also about finding out what the learners want to learn and how best they can learn it.

CREATING A LEARNING ENVIRONMENT

Learning can take place either formally or informally, and learning opportunities can be planned or they can just 'happen'. In both these situations, the effectiveness of the learning depends on the environment in which the learning takes place.

ACTIVITY 1
diary
Make some notes in your diary about what you think constitutes a good learning environment.

FEEDBACK

Points you may have noted include: providing somewhere suitable for you and the learner to meet; and making sure you have the time you need to cover everything properly and providing the right learning resources. Probably the most important factor in creating a successful learning environment is establishing a good relationship between the learner and the facilitator.

P6(i): Learning and communication explained the importance of communication between the learner and the facilitator in establishing the learner's needs. Becoming a facilitator involves adopting a certain frame of mind which puts the learner at the centre of the learning process. If the learning is to be effective, it is also important that the learner realises this: that it is the learner who is important, rather than you and what you want to get across.

For many people, especially those whose experience of learning has been dominated by traditional, formal methods, where they were told what they would learn, and then taught it and assessed as 'pass' or 'fail', this may take some getting used to.

ACTIVITY 2
diary
Think about how you would go about convincing someone who wants to learn that she is the most important factor in the learning process. What sorts of ideas would you want to get across? How might you express them?

FEEDBACK

Your answers to this Activity may have depended on who you had in mind, and your approach to this issue might well vary depending on whether you are dealing with students, clients or colleagues. However, in general, the most important points to get across to learners are that:

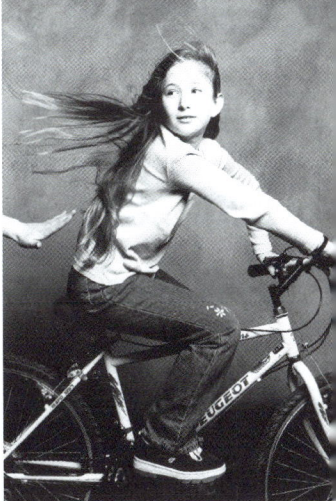

- Learning is a partnership. You are there to help, and if they do not understand, or have trouble learning something, it may be because you have not identified the right learning style for them, or because they have not expressed their learning needs clearly, rather than because they are incapable of learning

- Learning is a continuous process, not something to be dealt with in a session, but something to which you are happy to return in the future if the learners think it would help; for example: 'Try thinking it through for yourself afterwards, and then come back to me when you are clear about what you want to explore further'

- You expect and want the learners to express any worries they have, or any doubts or queries about what they are learning, and that you will always do your best to act on them.

If the learners concerned accept these points, and are comfortable with them, you will have created an environment in which the learning process is likely to be satisfactory for everyone.

THE FACILITATION PROCESS

Apart from communication, the most important issue in facilitating learning is structure. While the process of facilitation is focused on the learners, and their needs and wants, it helps if a simple structure is used to make sure that the learning takes place. The key features of the facilitation process may be listed as follows:

- Identifying a learning need

- Setting goals

- Identifying learning resources

- Planning and carrying out the facilitation

- Assessing and evaluating the learning.

These features do not always have to take place in this order, and some may take place at the same time as others.

Notes

Identifying a Learning Need

There are a number of different groups whose learning you may be able to facilitate. The Focus at the end of *P6(i): Learning and communication* asked you to use your skills of communication to find out the learning needs of two individuals *as they saw them.*

Once the learning need is identified, it is possible to move on to the next stage in the learning process.

Setting Goals

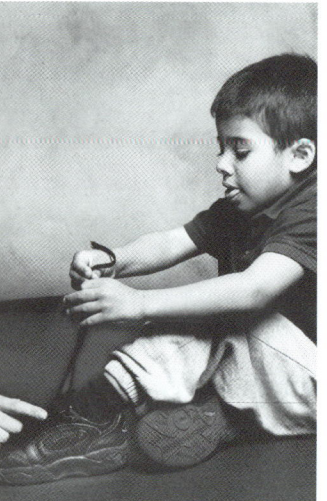

At the beginning of this programme, you worked with your tutor/counsellor to establish your own personal goals for the programme in response to your identified learning needs. Your experience of setting your own goals will help you to understand how other people carry out the process. This will make you a more effective facilitator of learning.

People may state their goals in a number of different ways.

EXAMPLES

- They may identify a skill which they want to develop, something which they could not do before, but which they want to learn; for example: 'I will learn how to take blood pressure'; 'I will learn how to recognise when I am becoming stressed'

- They may specify a new area of knowledge which they want to explore; for example: 'I want to find out more about attitudes to childbirth in certain ethnic communities', or 'I want to discover how other people of my age and social background have coped with the condition I am suffering from'

- They may state behavioural changes that they want to bring about; for example: 'I want to become a better time manager', or 'I want to cut down to four cigarettes a day'.

ACTIVITY 3
diary
Reflect on each of these different ways of expressing goals, and make some notes in your diary about what you think makes a good learning goal.

There are three key elements which make up a good learning goal:

- First, learners should be *clear* about what they want to achieve

- Second, you and the learners should both agree that the goal *can be achieved*

- Third, both you and the learners should have a way of assessing whether or not the goal has been achieved. This means that it must be *measurable.*

You may find that individual learners express their learning goals in one or more ways. As a facilitator you can work together to make sure that the learning goals are realistic.

Goal-setting is a vital exercise, both for learners and the facilitator. However, as you may have realised from your own experience of goal-setting, it can often be a case of agreeing what is possible rather than what is ideal. This may be particularly so with clients, where the reality of trying to change health-related behaviour is often an exercise in compromise. This is explored further in *P7: Health Promotion.*

Identifying Learning Resources

ACTIVITY 4
action
Choose one of the individuals whose learning needs you identified in the Focus in *P6(i): Learning and communication.* Carry out a goal-setting exercise based on his/her agreed learning needs. Make sure that the goals you agree on are clear, measurable, and achievable.

Learning resources can vary — they may, for example, be books, radio, newspapers, magazines, videos, journals or people. While some learning may take place through direct information-giving, it is important to remember that different people are motivated by different things, and learn in different ways. Variety, creativity and inspiration can all be important ingredients in successful learning.

ACTIVITY 5
action
Identify the main resources available for you to use to help other people to learn. The following list will start you off, but you will probably be able to add others. For each resource, say whether it is:
(a) present and an excellent learning resource
(b) present and a fair learning resource
(c) present and a poor learning resource
(d) not present.
• Staff in the clinical unit • Journal club • Staff in the community • Clients • Medical staff • Relatives • Paramedical staff • Friends • The public library • The local reference library • Books and articles • Evening classes • The nursing division of the university/college.
In the case of groups of people, you may not always be able to generalise about their quality as a learning resource. In this case, try to note any variations. For example, in the group 'medical staff', say why some are good learning resources and others poor.

FEEDBACK

You might find your answers to this Activity form the basis of a database of learning resources, to which you can add in the future.

Facilitating is about helping people to learn, but it doesn't necessarily mean you must always do it yourself. However, some nurses may feel that calling upon others, such as any one of the groups of people from the list in Activity 5, may undermine their own status as an 'expert'.

ACTIVITY 6
diary
How would you feel about using another person to facilitate learning with your colleagues or clients?

By drawing on the experience and knowledge of others, you may be able to reduce pressure on scarce resources, (that is, you!), and if the learning is effective, you have still been a facilitator, even if you weren't directly involved yourself.

Planning and Carrying Out the Facilitation

How these resources are used will depend on how you and the learners feel they will learn best. In this part of the process, you, as the facilitator, help the learners to plan how they will learn the new knowledge or skill identified as part of a learning need, and provide support as they work towards their goal.

How the learning goals are expressed will help you to determine the best use of the resources available to the learners. Goals relating to the acquisition of skills may need to be demonstrated by someone who has already mastered the skill, or the learners may need support as they try it for themselves. Such goals will almost always require a fairly high input of 'people' resources at least at some stage, if not throughout the whole process, and for this reason, skill development, especially of manual or technical skills, is often done as group work.

Different goals, different approaches

Goals which specify the acquisition of knowledge may demand a greater variety of resources. As explained at the start of the Research module, knowledge comes in many forms, and from many sources, and planning for this requires that all are used to best effect.

EXAMPLE

Finding out more about attitudes to childbirth in certain ethnic communities might require reading, discussion with health visitors or social workers, and discussion with members of the communities themselves, all of which, as you will know from your own experience on this programme, require planning and preparation if they are to be carried out successfully.

Goals which relate to changes in attitude or behaviour require yet another approach. The two main elements here will be information and support. Learners need to be as well-informed as possible about the choices available to them, and the implications of any change they make, and they also need to be supported as they make the necessary changes.

EXAMPLE

People who want to cut down on smoking need to be able to find out the possible methods by which they could do this, to be supported as they decide which is the best approach for them, and encouraged as they take the necessary steps to make the change.

You may find that you have to encourage the learners to break down a fairly large learning task into sub-goals, so that the whole process of learning becomes more manageable.

EXAMPLE

The goal of 'finding out more about mental illness' may involve the following actions:

- Borrowing a book about general psychiatry from the college library, and reading the introductory chapters

- Talking to a psychiatric nursing colleague about the differences between the various sorts of conditions

- Writing notes on the conditions, their treatments and nursing care

- Observing in clinical settings.

ACTIVITY 7
diary
Make some notes on the different ways each of the resources you identified in Activity 5 could be used. Which do you think would be the most appropriate to use in the case of the individual whose learning goals you agreed in Activity 4?

In planning how you are going to use these resources, you also need to bear in mind the time factor — your time and the learners' time. How able are the learners to find things out for themselves? Will you need to provide information in a more formal way? Make sure that you have the time, before you offer it.

Information-giving

As we have already indicated, facilitation does not just involve giving information. Although information-giving has its place in nursing and nurse education, facilitation is something different. It involves encouraging people to think things through and develop new ideas for themselves, with your support. Although you may find that you do supply information as part of the process, that is not an end in itself.

In the following table, two sets of situations are spelt out to show when information-giving may be appropriate, and when facilitation may be better.

INFORMATION-GIVING	FACILITATION
1. When advising a patient before surgery.	1. When talking through personal problems with a patient.
2. When giving a report or hand-over.	2. When helping a junior nurse to learn about physiology.
3. When conveying medical results to a colleague.	3. When organising clinical teaching.
4. When asked a direct question about side-effects of medication.	4. When helping a colleague to express emotion.

Learning which just 'happens'

ACTIVITY 8
diary
Identify two aspects of your own area of nursing that you feel would be best learnt by information-giving, and two that would be best learnt through facilitation. Make some notes in your diary explaining why.

Planning and carrying out the learning process are not separate, discrete items, or stages in the process that have an obvious beginning and end. Nor are they always easily recognisable. As we have seen, some of the most successful learning experiences just 'happen'. In fact, facilitating learning is often easiest when it happens by accident — when learners' interest is at its greatest, when the learning can be seen as directly relevant to what they are doing at present. However well you plan a learning programme, always remember that every nursing activity is a possible learning opportunity.

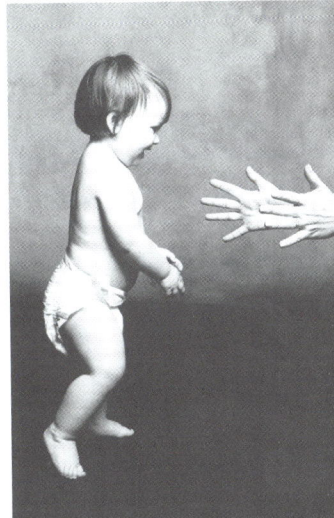

Assessing and Evaluating the Learning

However the learning takes place, the important last stage in the process is to consider how successful it has been. This involves two elements: *assessment* of the learners (whether they have achieved their goals) and *evaluation* of the learning process (how effective the learning was).

Just as planning and carrying out learning are not always a formal process, so assessment and evaluation often take place informally throughout the learning process rather than at the end of it.

As we saw earlier in this Part, assessing whether goals have been achieved is something which should be considered by both the facilitator and the learners. For example, if you have been helping learners to develop a new skill, they can be given the opportunity to show that they understand what needs to be done, that they can actually perform it, and that they have sought clarification of anything they are not sure about. In this case, both sides can agree that the goal has been achieved.

Other goals may be less straightforward to assess. The extent to which someone has changed behaviour is often a matter of opinion.

EXAMPLES

Although a goal such as 'cutting down to four cigarettes a day' is easily assessed, one like 'becoming a better time manager' is less clear-cut. In this case, learners must feel confident enough to make their own assessment without fear of being made to feel 'small' or inferior in any way because the facilitator does not agree with them.

ACTIVITY 9
diary

Can you remember any of your own learning experiences where assessment was delivered in a way that made you feel 'small', or a failure? Can you suggest how the way in which the assessment was delivered could have been done differently?

One way of avoiding damage to learners' self-esteem is to make it clear at the start of the learning process that it is important to you, the facilitator, that the learners achieve their goals, and that if they do not, it is just as likely to be because you have failed to agree the right approach or learning method as it is to any problem on the learners' part.

If the students accept this, they will be more likely to let you know when they do not understand something, or to suggest that you use a different approach which may be easier for them to understand.

Even if the learners have not learnt what they set out to learn, they should still be left with the feeling that they have gained something positive from the learning process — perhaps they discovered more about themselves, and identified new learning needs which they had not been aware of before. Perhaps they emerged with a clearer idea of themselves as learners, with a much better idea of how they would approach the same learning need next time. Perhaps the whole experience told them this was not an appropriate goal for them.

All of these are important outcomes of learning, even if the original goal was not right at the time. If the facilitator has created an environment in which feedback can be sought and given without the learners feeling that their self-esteem will be damaged by what they hear, then the facilitator will have been effective.

Taking this approach to assessment of the learners also helps you to evaluate the learning process itself. The feedback you get will give you a feel for how successful you have been in helping the learners to learn. However, you might also want to ask some specific questions at the end of the process — open questions which give the learners plenty of scope to express their feelings, rather than tell you what they think you want to hear. It is at this stage that the effectiveness of the learning environment you have created will bring benefits to you as well as to the learners.

What If It Hasn't Worked?

If the learning plan has not been successful, that is, if the students or clients have not acquired the knowledge, skills or understanding that they wanted to, then you need to take the evaluation a stage further and find out why.

Many factors can get in the way of learning. You may already have been able to identify from feedback a fault in the learning programme itself, or in your own approach to facilitation. In this case, you may need to go back to the beginning of the process and start again.

Other things, too, may prevent people from learning. These might include:

- Tiredness

- Fear of failure

- Pressure of work

- Lack of confidence as a learner

- Making unfavourable comparisons with other people

- Conflicting things happening at the time.

How much can you as a facilitator do about any of these problems? The self-esteem issue is an important one, and the right sort of learning environment, as discussed at the start of this Part, will do a great deal to maintain and enhance learners' self-esteem.

Assessment and evaluation complete the facilitation process although, as we have seen, they often both go on throughout, rather than just at the end. From identifying needs, you have worked through to finding out whether the needs have been met. Now the process can start again. It is invariably the case that one learning project leads on to another.

FOCUS

How do you rate yourself as a facilitator? Think of an occasion in the past, either in your personal or professional life, when you have helped someone to learn something.

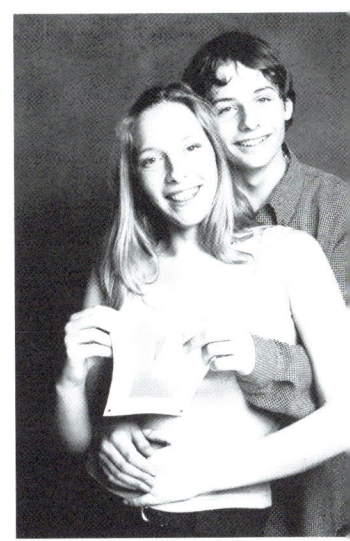

Make some notes on:

- Whether you think you were a successful facilitator on this occasion

- What you might do differently now

- What areas you would like to develop to become a better facilitator in the future.

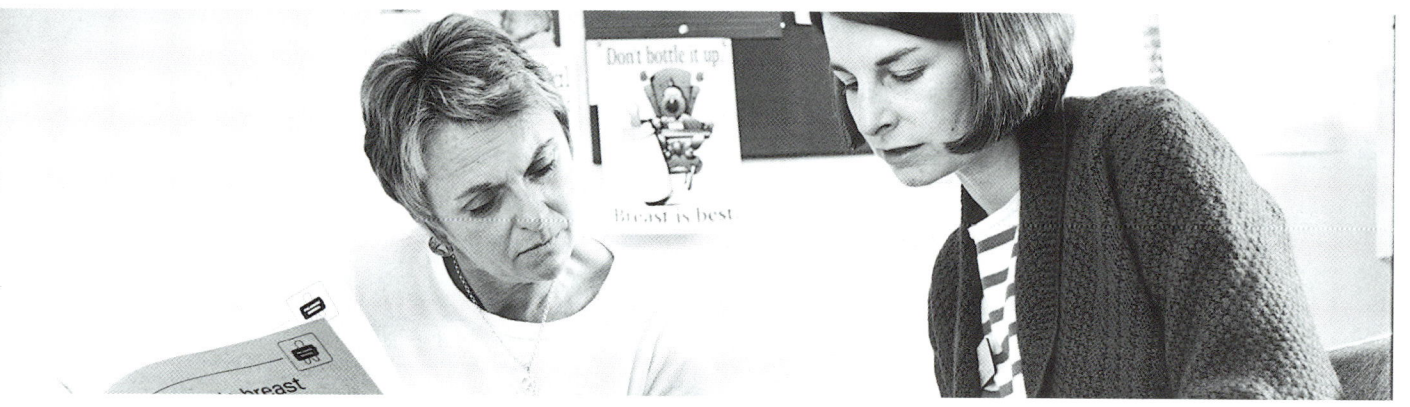

Health promotion: a question of choice?

The three Parts in *P7: Health Promotion,* look at the impact that health promotion has on our profession. Here you will examine the factors which influence people's decisions about health, and explore ways in which the health promoter can help to make those decisions healthy ones for each individual client or patient.

Points covered include:

- The state of Britain's health as discussed in the Black Report
- Whether health should be a party political issue
- The major factors which influence individual decisions about health
- Different models of health promotion
- Health promotion in your own practice
- The amount of control individuals have over issues which affect their health.

WORK PLANNER

Your work on health promotion will focus on individuals — their attitudes to their own health, and to you as a health promoter. This will build on work you may have already completed on attitudes to health in *P1: Health and Illness, P2: Human Biography* and *P5: Client Assessment.* You may wish to review these briefly before starting.

In Activity 1, you are asked to look at a copy of P. Townsend's and N. Davidson's book *Inequalities in Health: The Black Report*, published by Penguin Books (1982), and which should be available in your college library.

Activity 3 asks you to monitor the coverage of health issues in the news media over the period of a week. You may want to set yourself a reminder to catch the news and look at one or two newspapers over this period.

Activity 5 asks you to make contact with your local health promotion unit and arrange to meet one of the health promoters there. You will find the address of your local unit and the names of possible contacts through your local council's Department of Public Health. You may want to arrange your visit now, before you begin work on this Part.

Activity 7 suggests discussion with students from other practice areas. You may want to look out for an opportunity at this stage and make a firm arrangement to meet.

You might also wish to look at the unit on health promotion from the Emap Healthcare Open Learning BSc (Hons) Professional Practice in Health Care — *Health Promotion in Professional Practice* (see the Introduction to this book, page 3, for details on how to obtain a copy).

A HEALTHY NATION?

P4(iii): Acquiring level-1 competences introduced the King's Fund concept of health promotion[1], which argued that health promotion implies two levels of action: a *policy* level and an *individual* level.

At the *policy* level, governments and public authorities decide on policy, laws and economic strategies which they believe will enhance rather than hinder the population's health.

EXAMPLES

Encouraging the use of lead-free petrol by introducing subsidies; providing public education programmes; and restrictions on oil companies and car manufacturers, with the aim of reducing air pollution are all examples of health promotion at the policy level.

In addition, there are many laws or policies which, at first sight, may not seem to be directly related to the population's health.

EXAMPLES

Transport, agriculture and industrial expansion can all be indirectly related to health promotion issues.

As explained in *P3(i): Public health and personal health*, there is an enormous body of legislation about public health.

At the *individual* level of action, health promotion is concerned with people and communities enjoying better health through informed self-care, self-help and changing behaviour towards healthier life-styles.

In reality, it is impossible to separate these two aspects. The health of the nation is the product of individual decisions about health made by every member of the population, and much of what individuals do is shaped by government action.

Government policies on housing, unemployment benefit and occupational health have just as much influence on the health of individuals as do the policies to promote health that we mentioned above.

The Black Report

The Black Report[2] in 1980 pointed out the effect of socio-economic factors on health, concluding that Britain was still 'two nations' in terms of health. It showed that, although the health of the nation as a whole had improved in the 30 years since the formation of the NHS, the gap between the health of professional and skilled groups in society and that of manual and unskilled groups had, in fact, widened.

The Black Report recommendations were never implemented, and the continued existence of the social disparities that it noted were discussed in the King's Fund report on the nation's health[1]. It could be argued that a clear opportunity to improve the nation's health had been missed.

Health and Party Politics

ACTIVITY 1
action
Spend some time looking at the Summary and Recommendations of the Black Report, and read in more detail any sections which are of particular interest to your own area of practice.

Health promotion has become a topical issue. A variety of people have contributed to this, including the former junior minister in the Department of Health from 1986–1988, Edwina Currie. You may remember her controversial remarks about the diet of northerners, and her role in the salmonella-in-eggs crisis. A politician who comments about health promotion issues and loses her job clearly emphasises to the public the *political* nature of health promotion.

In the current White Paper, *The New NHS: Modern, Dependable*[3], there is an emphasis on health promotion and prevention rather than cure. Through Health Action Zones and the Health Improvement Programme, the government seeks to bring together all professionals and organisations that are involved in improving the quality of life of people — and their health-related needs. So, for example, nurses will now be encouraged to work alongside housing officers and social services staff to target improving the lives of elderly people living in inappropriate accommodation.

ACTIVITY 2
diary
Do you think health promotion should be a high-profile political issue? Reflect on some of the benefits and dangers of involving party politics in health promotion. Make a few notes in your diary.

FEEDBACK

You may have thought that politicians who pronounce on health issues hinder rather than help those who are actually involved in health promotion. It might be better if politicians tried, for example, to change government subsidies, rather than making some groups in society feel guilty or resentful about their life-styles.

Alternatively, you may have felt that 'there is no such thing as bad publicity' — that anyone or anything that makes people more aware of health issues is better than nothing at all.

The politics of health promotion is much wider, however, than party politics. It extends to issues such as attitudes to mental health and illness, the role of women, the rights of children and the influence of the profit motive in guiding consumer choice.

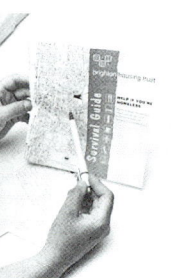
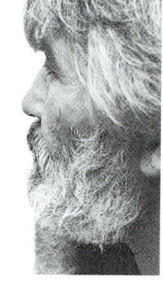

ACTIVITY 3
action
As you work through *P7: Health Promotion*, reflect on the ways in which public policy and individual health decisions are linked. Over the next week, monitor coverage of health issues in the news media, and make some notes on how the viewpoints of various interested groups are represented.

HEALTH DECISIONS

As we said above, the health of the nation is the product of all the health decisions made by each member of society. As the Black Report indicated, public policy influences these decisions in many ways, but it is just one of the range of factors that determine each individual decision.

The following diagram illustrates the major factors which affect individual decisions about health.

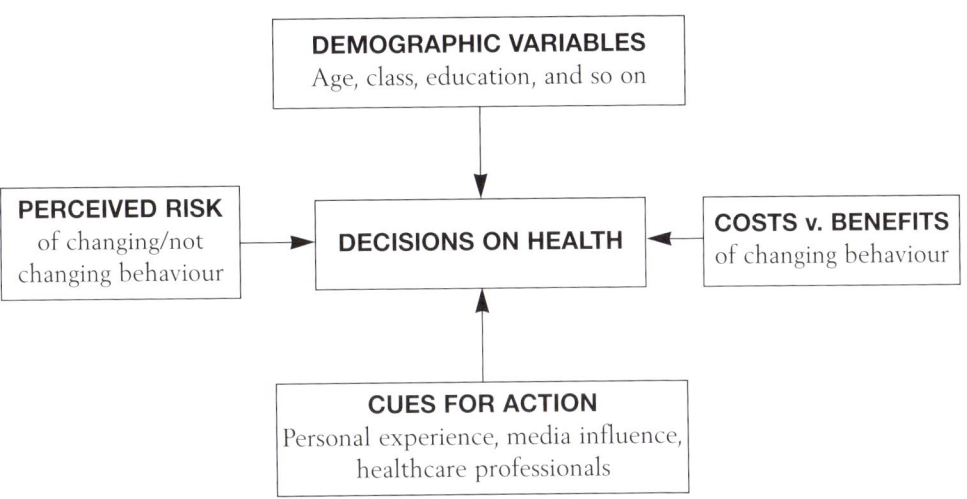

Health decisions are taken by each individual weighing up the health risk as he/she sees it in a particular course of action, and assessing the costs and benefits to them of such an action.

Of course, people do not usually go through this procedure consciously. Much of the knowledge on which their decisions are based is the mutual knowledge of their own particular social group and they tend to behave in a particular way because most of the other people they know also behave in that way.

People are also influenced, either consciously or unconsciously, by other forms of knowledge — personal experience is a major influence, as is the culture in which they live, and other external sources, such as media and advertising.

EXAMPLE

Although smoking is on the decline in the population as a whole, it is declining less quickly among women. There are also increasing numbers of young people who smoke, and evidence shows that health promotion campaigns over the past 10 years have not yet tackled this issue successfully.

Let's take another example — alcohol consumption.

ACTIVITY 4
diary
List the factors you think influence people's decision about whether and why to drink alcohol.

FEEDBACK

Whether we drink alcohol or not is influenced by many factors, such as:

- **Age** — we probably drink most in our twenties

- **Gender** — females tend to consume different types of drinks than males do, and in some cultures tend to have their drinks bought for them

- **Money** — will influence whether it is an expensive whisky or meths we are drinking

- **Legislation** — the licensing laws and taxes determine the price. The government received £200 every second in 1986 from taxes on alcohol and, incidentally, spent 0.1 pence per second on alcohol education and therapy

- **Religion** — alcohol is banned in some religions

- **Culture** and **class**

- **Occupation** — in some jobs alcohol is freely available

- **Feasts** and **celebrations**

- Being **happy** or **sad**

- Being **sociable**, or because our peers indulge

- Because we **like it**
- Our **family background** and **family role**
- **Personality**
- **Advertising**

These examples illustrate the range of factors which can influence people's conscious or unconscious health decisions. We will now begin to explore how health promoters fit into the picture by examining what we mean by health promotion, and some of the ways we can go about it in practice.

WHAT IS HEALTH PROMOTION?

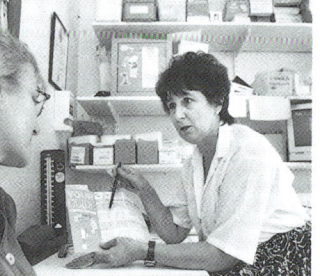

The term health promotion is a fairly new one. In 1984 the World Health Organization (WHO) began a programme of discussions about health promotion, and concluded that the idea has come to represent 'a unifying concept for those who recognise the need for change in the ways and conditions of living, in order to promote health'. It links people and their environments, and balances personal choice and social responsibility in health to create a healthier future.

In more recent years there have been a number of influential reports outlining the importance of health promotion. You might like to read:

- Hills, D. and King, A. *Meeting the Targets or Meeting the Community*. A discussion paper from the Tavistock Institute Review, 1994

- Naidoo, J. and Wills, J. *Health promotion: Foundations for practice*. London: Bailliere Tindall, 1994

- Robson, C. *Real World Research*. Oxford: Blackwell, 1993.

Promoting better health covers a wide spectrum of activities for nurses, and we can use three different models to consider how we approach these activities.

The Preventive, or Behaviour Change Approach

This is the traditional model of health education, based on a medical view of health problems. It is geared towards preventing illness, rather than promoting well-being or health in its widest sense. This approach tends to be 'expert-led'; that is, the healthcare expert hands down the advice, and the public, clients or patients make their decisions based on what they are told.

We can think of this approach in terms of primary, secondary and tertiary prevention measures.

Primary prevention is concerned with preventing disease, disability and premature death occurring in the first place, and includes such measures as immunisation programmes, 'safer sex' campaigns and seat-belt legislation.

Secondary prevention takes place when an illness has occurred, and educational strategies are used to restore the person to full health, or to prevent the condition becoming chronic or irreversible. This might include measures such as helping a person with diabetes comply with medical advice, or a patient with heart problems stop smoking and reduce weight.

Tertiary prevention occurs when a complete cure cannot be achieved, or there is some permanent impairment, as in the case of strokes, amputation or colostomy. The emphasis here is very much on rehabilitation, preventing complications, and helping and educating patients, their partners and their relatives to make the most of their remaining potential for healthy living.

Self-empowerment

This approach to health promotion focuses on encouraging people to believe that they are in charge of their own lives. Although much of the information involved might be the same as in the approach we discussed above, this approach, rather than 'handing down' information from experts, encourages the development of self-esteem, life skills, assertiveness, and so on.

Social Change

The social change approach to health promotion focuses on the idea that social, economic and political factors have a major impact on health. It promotes activities which aim to change social or environmental policy, either at local or national level. Although, again, it may involve similar information, this is a 'bottom-up' approach, rather than the 'top down' approach of our first model. Some examples would include introducing a no-smoking policy in the workplace, or creating local pressure to reduce dog excreta in public places.

ACTIVITY 5
action

Make contact with your local health promotion unit and arrange to meet one of the health promotion advisers. Explain that you would like to meet someone with whom you can discuss ideas and problems relating to health promotion.
The unit might have its own library. While you are there, take a look at the resources available — videos and teaching packs — and make a list of any you might find useful in your own area of practice.
After your visit, make some notes in your diary of the points and issues raised at your meeting.

WHICH APPROACH IS BEST?

As we have said, each of these approaches can involve the same information. What differs in each case is how the information is 'sold', and how the individual is encouraged to act on that information.

ACTIVITY 6
diary

Think about a specific health promotion issue which is important in your own practice, and about the type of information which would promote better health in that area.
Which of the above approaches do you currently use to get this information across to those who need it?

FEEDBACK

In practice, all the approaches discussed have a role to play in health promotion, and you may have found in answering the previous Activity that the boundaries between them are not particularly clear-cut. However, it may also have prompted you to reflect that some approaches may be more appropriate than others in particular situations.

ACTIVITY 7
discussion

If you have a chance to meet students from other practice areas, compare answers to the previous Activity and consider why they might be different in different types of practice.

Perhaps the most important thing to emerge from these last two Activities is that most of us will find that we are already doing quite a lot of health promotion, even though we might not have given it such a label. Can we, by identifying 'health promotion' as a distinctive part of our responsibilities, improve on what we already do?

169

READY TO CHANGE?

We have explored some of the factors which influence individual decisions about health, and have considered different ways in which the activity of promoting health might be approached. But how do we actually change people's behaviour?

A 1983 survey on health behaviour among the general population[4] found that 47% of British people had improved their lifestyle by, for example, changing their diet, taking more exercise, or relaxing more, all of their own accord, without any direct prompting from GPs or nurses. So it would seem that there is a fair amount of scope to achieve even more than this if healthcare professionals are directly involved.

It is now the case that our calorie intake is around 20% less than 10 years ago, so the health promotion campaign on diet has been successful. However, it is equally true that the number of people dying from heart disease is rising. This is because most of us get less exercise than we need — we use the car to go to the shops and we watch more TV; generally, our life-style is more sedentary.

Nurses have proved that they can be successful in promoting healthier lifestyles. In a very difficult area to change — smoking reduction — nurses undergoing a short training course found that they could achieve a 17% reduction in smoking with their clients,[5] and in America, nurses found that even after a three-minute teaching session with patients in hospital, the patients began to choose healthier foods from the menu[6].

There are many factors, both within nursing and in the public eye, which have brought more pressure for nurses to be competent health promoters.

ACTIVITY 8
diary
Can you think of any issues or events which have made health promotion more important for nurses in the 1990s? List them in your diary.

FEEDBACK

Some of the issues you could have listed include:

- The increase once again this century of infectious diseases, particularly AIDS, but also others such as Legionnaire's disease

- The growing realisation that modern, high-tech medicine cannot meet all our needs

- Demand for improved quality of life, arising out of issues such as the safety of food: salmonella in chickens and eggs; listeria in soft cheeses; radiation in sheep affected by the Chernobyl disaster; 'mad cow' disease (BSE) in meat, sausages and pies; hormones in factory-farmed pigs and salmon; lead in our vegetables; mercury in seafood; E coli bacteria in meat

- The change in illness patterns — many of today's diseases are very suitable targets for health promotion: cancers, circulatory problems, stress, environmental and pollution hazards

- The changing role of the nurse — nurses are keen to develop and expand their role into teaching and research, and to develop nursing as a profession in its own right

- Consumer demand: patients today require nurses to have communication and assessment skills, knowledge, and an ability to analyse

- Project 2000. This approach to the training of nurses recognises the changes in society and correspondingly requires nurses also to develop.

There is pressure, therefore, from many sources for us to be more effective health promoters. The other parts of *P7: Health Promotion*, explore how we can do this. However, we end this Part by questioning how far we as nurses can go to change people's behaviour.

How Much Control Do We Have?

We have referred to the notion of control several times in this Part, and have described health decisions in terms of a rational (or sometimes irrational) response by individuals to certain information which is made publicly available through various channels, including healthcare professionals.

Let's take the example of choices about food, to explore how much control an individual has.

EXAMPLE

You are able to limit the amount of saturated fat you take in from milk if your local shop is able to supply skimmed milk, but you have no control over the BST (bovine somatotrophin) in the milk (put there to increase the yield); the BSE crisis raised issues about the feed given to cattle and its possible effects on humans who eat meat. The water we drink often comes with worms and larvae, not to mention bacteria and viruses. We are not able individually to influence this, unless we are prepared to spend money on bottled water.

Other factors also serve to limit the amount of individual choice we have about health. For example, a family's income will influence the type of food they are able to buy, as will things like accessibility to shops for old people, or those in rural areas.

Finally, culture and class also influence the choice and availability of certain types of food. Some people eat a lot of fried foods, whereas others eat many more salad foods.

ACTIVITY 9
diary
How much control do you think you have over the food you eat? In your diary, draw a line like the one below and mark on it an X to indicate where you think your control lies. Then repeat the exercise for two or three of your patients or clients.

This exercise shows that, while there are some factors over which individuals can exercise control, there are many others over which they can have little influence as individuals.

Complete control _____ No control

You may want to repeat this exercise for other factors, such as the amount of control we have over the environment in which we live.

FOCUS

Look back over the work you have done in this Part and reflect on your own views on health promotion in your own practice. Make a note of opportunities you can identify for additional health promotion. Were there any resources at the health promotion unit you visited which you would now use?

Consider what has prevented you from actively promoting health in the past, and note down any worries and dilemmas that you might have. You may want to discuss these points with your tutor/counsellor.

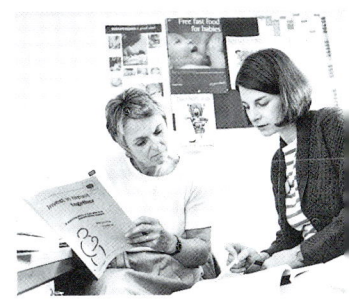

Notes   REFERENCES

1   The King's Fund. *The Nation's Health: A strategy for the 1990s.* London: The King's Fund, 1988.

2   Townsend, P., Davidson, N. *Inequalities in Health: The Black Report.* Harmondsworth: Penguin Books, 1982.

3   Department of Health. *The New NHS: Modern, Dependable.* London: The Stationery Office, Cmnd 3807, 1997.

4   Anderson, R. How have people changed their health behaviour? *Health Education Journal* 1983; **42**: 3, 82–86.

5   MacLeod, Clark, J., Kendall, S., Haverty, S. *Helping People to Stop Smoking: The nurse's role.* London: Health Education Authority, 1979.

6   Packard, R. B., Van Ess, H. A comparison of informal and role-delineated patient teaching situations. *Nursing Research* 1969; **18**: 5; 443–444.

FURTHER READING

•   Department of Health. *The Health of the Nation: A strategy for health in England.* London: HMSO, 1992.

•   Ewles, L., Simnett, I. *Promoting Health: A practical guide.* London: Scutari Press, 1992.

•   LeTouze, S. and Calnan, M. Health promotion in general practice: The views of staff. *Nursing Times* 1996; **92**: 1, 32–33.

•   Tannahill, A. Health education and health promotion planning for the 1990s. *Health Education Journal* 1990; **49**: 194–198.

•   Whitehead, M., Tones, B. *Avoiding the Pitfalls.* London: Health Education Authority, 1991.

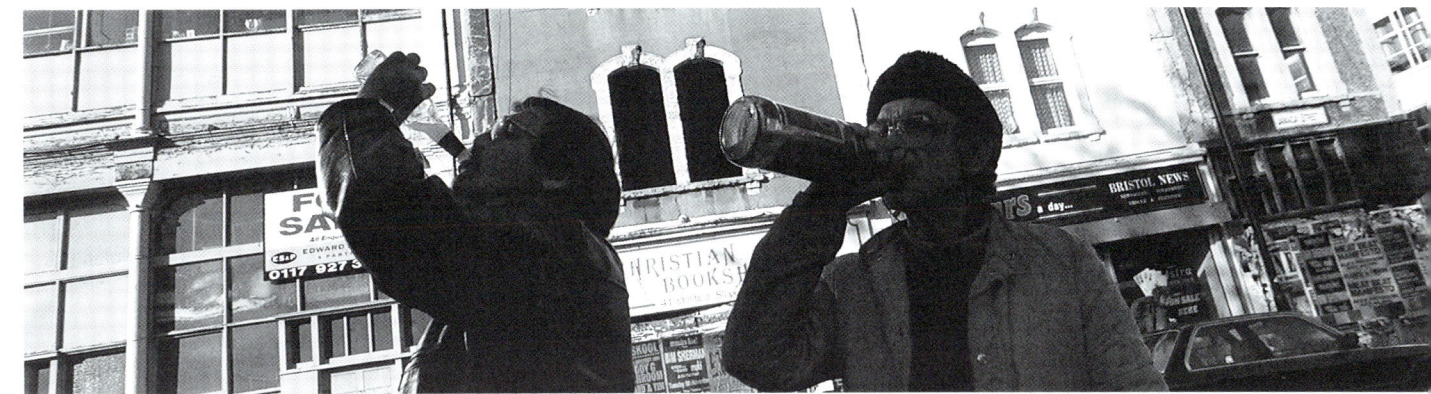

Issues and dilemmas

Active health promotion is about changing people's behaviour. Many nurses have problems with this — problems relating to their own confidence, and unease about interfering in other people's lives.

The end of *P7(i): Health Promotion: A question of choice?* asked you to identify some of the issues and dilemmas which might prevent you from promoting health as effectively as you would like. Here you will look at some of these problem areas, and, it is to be hoped, find some solutions which work for you. You will focus on:

* How much do I tell?

* Is my knowledge good enough?

* What if I advise someone to do something that proves to be harmful?

* How persuasive can I be?

* Is it right for me to try to change social behaviour?

* Am I a good role model?

WORK PLANNER

This Part includes practical ways in which you can increase your knowledge about health promotion issues. You may find it helpful to re-read *R1: Nursing: A research-based profession.*

Activity 8 asks you to start a system for expanding your health promotion knowledge. You may want to look ahead to this to schedule enough time for undertaking it.

If you would like to explore the subject of health promotion further, the unit entitled *Health Promotion in Professional Practice* from the Emap Healthcare Open Learning BSc (Hons) Professional Practice in Health Care may be useful as it contains a wealth of references on the subject (see the Introduction to this book, page 3, for details on how to obtain a copy).

A QUESTION OF APPROACH

We start this Part by looking at a case study which provides a number of opportunities for health promotion.

CASE STUDY

Sylvia Clarke is 62 years old and married. During a family gathering she had a minor heart attack and was admitted to the coronary care unit where she subsequently had another more major infarction, plus more cardiac complications. Two-and-a-half weeks later she was admitted to a general medical ward.

Mrs Clarke lives with her 63-year-old husband in local authority housing in Ashton-under-Lyne. They have three children, two in their late thirties and the oldest 44, and seven grandchildren ranging in age from four to 18. Before she retired, Mrs Clarke worked in a clothing factory where her husband still works.

Neither of them has enjoyed particularly good health and both of them have smoked. Mr Clarke gave up eight years ago, but Mrs Clarke still smokes occasionally. She is slightly overweight and also has occasional dizzy spells.

Mrs Clarke is a lively, friendly, out-going person who is always talking. She has had a tremendous fright from this recent experience and is looking forward to going home soon.

What follows are two caricature profiles of nurses who each take a very different approach towards Mrs Clarke. These are extreme responses to the situation, but aspects of both behaviours do occur.

Staff Nurse Feather Duster's approach: one approach is the staff nurse who says she does not really approve of delving into people's private lives and telling them how to behave. She is able to identify some areas where a change to a healthier way of life would be beneficial for Mrs Clarke, but feels her role is to concentrate on helping her patient recover from the heart attack. This nurse tends to chat a lot about resting, and not worrying, and about keeping cheerful and looking on the bright side. No mention is ever made of changing Mrs Clarke's diet and reducing saturated fat intake, or about her eating more fruit and vegetables, less red meat and meat products, more fibre-rich foods and fewer refined carbohydrates.

This nurse also does not bother to mention how lack of exercise and a sedentary way of life can be harmful. She is aware of research evidence which suggests that go-getting, competitive personalities such as Mrs Clarke's might contribute to heart attacks, but is not sure what can be done about that anyway.

Smoking is an activity which this nurse knows definitely contributes to heart attacks, but feels that Mrs Clarke might be offended, or that she might worry, if the subject is brought up. Anyway, she feels that it is too late to try and change Mrs Clarke's habit now.

Mrs Clarke's blood pressure is usually high, but there is no problem there: Staff Nurse Feather-Duster is able to give her some tablets to keep it low.

Preparation for home, Nurse Feather-Duster knows, is an area where good planning is essential. The district nurse needs to be asked to call to help with washes, the patient's GP will be informed by the doctor's summary letter (eventually) and a follow-up appointment should be booked. Drugs to take home are ready and waiting, as is the booklet which talks about lifting and resuming sexual relations.

Staff Nurse Sledge-Hammer's approach: A more direct, aggressive approach is taken by a second type of staff nurse. Her first health promotion aim is to stop the patient smoking. She feels that the means justify the ends, and that ultimately it is for Mrs Clarke's own good. Diet and exercise and, finally, stress reduction, are all approached in the same way.

Each topic is taken with the same determination and confidence: 'It's up to you, you know, Mrs Clarke. I can only give you the facts. If you want to go on eating saturated fats, it will be your funeral, not mine.'

'Well, Mrs Clarke, do you want to die? Or do you want to live? Now I'm confiscating all these remaining cigarettes, and I want you to promise that this will be the end of all this smoking.'

HOW MUCH DO I TELL?

ACTIVITY 1
diary
Make some notes in your diary about your opinions of the approaches of these two nurses to their patient's needs. How successful do you think they will be? Can you recognise any aspects of your own behaviour in these caricatures?

One of the major dilemmas nurses are faced with is exactly *how much* to tell their patients. Nowadays, most people are fairly well-informed about health issues and expect their professional carers to tell them almost everything and, up to a certain point, most nurses would agree with this. The days are gone when the debate was about whether or not to tell patients their diagnosis — now the issue is more likely to be *how* to tell them.

ACTIVITY 2
diary
Can you think of any incidents in your professional career (a) where you thought that information was withheld from a patient; (b) where a patient was told too much? Make some notes in your diary, giving reasons for your views.

Both these situations can and do arise, and there are no hard and fast rules about what to tell. Each situation requires you to use your communication skills to determine the needs of your patient. Some people will want to know everything about their condition, and the way you are treating it. In such cases it is your responsibility to inform them in a sensitive manner which is direct and straightforward, so that they believe they are being told everything. Others will not want to know so much and you will need to move at their pace to determine exactly what they require.

Surveys indicate that between 30 and 60% of patients are dissatisfied with explanations, information and advice given to them by doctors and that, generally, most people benefit from as much information as possible. Research work has indicated that telling, in a sensitive and caring way, helps most patients and, where relevant, their carers in the community, to cope best with their situation[1,2].

ACTIVITY 3
diary
Mrs Clarke, from the case study above, wants to know: 'Why do you suppose I had this heart attack, Nurse? The doctor tells me it was rather a serious one and I'm really worried that I may have another one. Do you think I will?' Write down what you think the two caricature nurses would have said. Would your own reply have any elements from one or the other?

The second nurse in the two examples would have all the information at her fingertips and would tell Mrs Clarke straightaway that about 35% of people who have had a heart attack and who make it to hospital do in fact die, but that if she survives the first month then Mrs Clarke has a 50–50 chance of being alive five years later.

The more hesitant nurse would tell Mrs Clarke that everything was fine and to look on the bright side.

ACTIVITY 4
diary
Now think carefully about how to take a positive approach and be realistic at the same time. What are the important factors in replying to a question such as that given by Mrs Clarke in the previous Activity?

When answering patients' questions, the first thing you need to do is to acknowledge their worries and confirm that they are valid. At the same time you need to provide some concrete help on improving their health and promoting a healthier lifestyle. To do this you need to find out what they understand about their condition so that you don't waste time explaining something they know already.

The problem about how much information to divulge occurs in every specialty within nursing, and may be one of the things preventing us from embarking upon health promotion.

EXAMPLE

The nurse working with patients with mental health problems may have to face the dilemma of how to explain the effects and side-effects of some treatments; the health visitor may have to decide whether to persuade mothers to have the whooping cough vaccine for their babies, knowing that the whooping cough vaccination programme has been abandoned in Sweden because of uncertainties about the safety of one particular vaccine[3]; and a nurse working with patients having radiotherapy may face difficulties in deciding how much emphasis to place on explaining the negative aspects of the treatment.

> **ACTIVITY 5**
> **diary**
> Identify a patient or a situation in which you were involved where health promotion was less than honest because of the dilemma of how much to tell. Make some brief notes on how the interaction could have been improved.

IS MY KNOWLEDGE GOOD ENOUGH?

This is a worry which often inhibits us from embarking upon health promotion: the fear that we don't know enough.

> **ACTIVITY 6**
> **diary**
> Think of an occasion from your own practice where you held back from giving advice on health because you felt your knowledge was insufficient. Did you take any action to remedy the situation?

CASE STUDY

Debbie was a newly qualified staff nurse working in a children's ward in a large teaching hospital. She noticed that two of her patients, although similar in age, were very different in their use of language. Both the girls were four years old and one of them kept asking her questions; so many, in fact, that Debbie decided to count them — in one hour she was asked 90 questions. On the other hand, the other girl asked only three questions.

Debbie was worried that this language variation might be a cause for concern, but she did not know which pattern was the healthy one.

> **ACTIVITY 7**
> **diary**
> How do you think Debbie could find out what is 'normal' behaviour for a four-year-old? Make some notes in your diary about how you might approach this situation.

FEEDBACK

The first step to take would be to talk to an experienced paediatric nurse, who would see that it is quite normal for four-year-olds to be asking questions all the time. The experienced nurse would probably suggest to Debbie that she should read a research report on this.

Research carried out by Barbara Tizard and Martin Hughes, which examined tape-recorded conversations between mothers and four-year-olds and the same children and their nursery school teachers, found an enormous variation in the amount of questioning a happy, relaxed child, who was intent on discovery, would engage in[4]. The average number was 45 questions an hour; however, some very bright children asked up to 140 questions.

Concern might therefore be for the child who asked only a few questions.

Expanding my Knowledge of Health Promotion

We all have gaps in our knowledge — no one can know everything. What is important is the action we take to remedy the situation. In R2(i) and R2(ii), you examined your existing network of knowledge resources, and explored some techniques for expanding and enhancing your nursing knowledge. Health promotion is one of the areas where you can use these techniques in practice.

ACTIVITY 8
knowledge base

Look back at *R2(ii): Rubbing shoulders with research* which explored the various media and people through which research-based knowledge is disseminated.
For each of the types of source listed, identify those which provide health promotion information in your specialty. Consider in general terms the sort of information your clients need, and where the gaps in your knowledge lie.
You may want to start a special file (card index) for 'Health Promotion', and add to it whenever you read or hear about something you think might help in the future.

Try to keep a separate person as a mentor for health promotion. You could possibly use the health promotion adviser based at your nearest health promotion unit, or a clinical nurse specialist, a nurse researcher or a tutor with an interest in the topic.

ACTIVITY 9
action

Try to identify a person with whom you could liaise for up-to-date information on health promotion issues. Then do so.

The next dilemma which can interfere with our ability to give good health promotion is one which Staff Nurse Feather-Duster knows a lot about, and Staff Nurse Sledge-Hammer should think more about.

WHAT IF I ADVISE SOMEONE TO DO SOMETHING WHICH PROVES TO BE HARMFUL?

This is a fear about taking full responsibility for your professional actions. You engage in many physical activities for your patients which may prove to be harmful: giving them medications, taking them for radiotherapy or surgery, even giving them enemas and changing their dressings. You are confident that you know how to do these things, and you try your best not to harm them in the physical care you provide. It follows that if you are sure of the soundness of the knowledge on which your advice is based, you will do the same for psychological care and health promotion. The more you know and understand about your nursing knowledge base, the less likely it is that you will offer inaccurate advice.

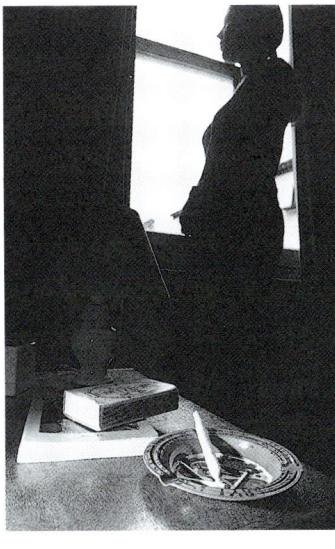

EXAMPLE

Diet and nutrition are areas where there has been a lot of inconclusive information and some conflicting research data. Do additives and colourings influence behaviour in children? Will vitamin supplements enhance their IQ? Do patients in psychiatric hospitals have a nutrient-deficient diet and does this affect their recovery? What about the government's healthy eating advice, and the relationships between diet and cancer?

ACTIVITY 10
diary
What advice do you offer the patients or clients in your area of work about diet and nutrition? Make some notes in your diary.

FEEDBACK

If you don't offer any advice, is it because you are uncertain about its validity? One way of overcoming this is to keep up to date, using the methods we discussed in Activity 8, and discuss as often as possible all new research findings with colleagues. This will not only help you update your own knowledge base, but ensure that all colleagues are giving the same information to clients.

HOW PERSUASIVE CAN I BE? IS IT RIGHT FOR ME TO TRY TO CHANGE SOCIAL BEHAVIOUR?

Many nurses are reticent about talking to their patients about personal habits such as eating, smoking or sexual behaviour, as they feel that it is none of their business. They feel that as long as the patients have the facts about the health risks of their behaviour, it is ultimately up to them to change if they want to. Yet as nurses we also know that it has been well established that some social behaviours can lead to harmful outcomes, and most people do, in fact, want help in changing behaviour which harms them. It is our responsibility to raise the issue, and if patients wish to change a harmful behaviour then we need to find a suitable method of helping them.

Consider what methods are available to you to do this.

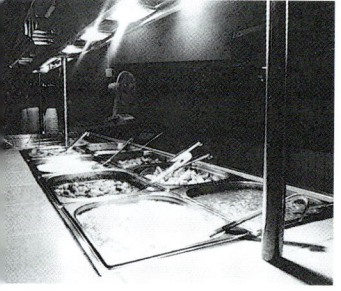

ACTIVITY 11
diary
If you were in the position to withhold an expensive resource (such as surgery) from a patient who was unable to give up smoking, would you? Would you use the threat of withholding it in an attempt to get the patient to change this habit?

FEEDBACK

How we answer questions such as this may depend upon our own beliefs and values. As explained in earlier Sections, if our own feelings about a subject differ from those of our clients, we may fail to convey or interpret information in the most appropriate way for them.

EXAMPLE

There are two possible perspectives on safer sex — that the only way is to have one stable partner, or that the number of partners doesn't matter, as long as you practise safer sex with them all. If you believe the second of these perspectives to be morally wrong, this might affect the sort of health promotion you provide.

Another belief that might influence your approach to health promotion is the belief that we are all free to make our own health choices.

The term 'freedom of choice' is one that you will have heard quite a bit about in relation to health promotion. As health promoters, we say we want to help people make their own choices. However, as we saw last week, freedom of choice is often just a myth. McKeown[5] gives us this example:

'Our habits commonly begin as pleasures of which we have no need, and end as necessities in which we have no pleasure. Nevertheless we tend to resent the suggestion that any one should try to change them, even on the disarming grounds that they do so for our own good ... It is said that the individual must be free to choose whether he wishes to smoke. But he is not free; with a drug of addiction the option is open only at the beginning, so that the critical decision to smoke is taken, not by consenting adults but by children below the age of consent.'

ACTIVITY 12
diary
Identify someone from your personal life — a friend or relative — who you think lacks control over a harmful health-related activity and make some notes about the methods you would use to help this person change the situation.

To return to your nursing life now, the best approach with clients or patients lies in finding a way of persuading them to take responsibility for their own decisions, based on information and advice from you. You will have more chance of succeeding in this if you include the following in your approach:

- Provide patients with facts and information and make sure that they completely understand all the issues. This may take quite a lot of time, which will have to be planned for

- Identify and help patients come to terms with some of the emotions that this knowledge brings. For example, a patient brought up in the Asian community, who uses a lot of butter in food, and who needs lose weight, may experience some emotional difficulty when changing dietary habits as he may feel that it distances him from his culture

- Give the patient the opportunity to practise decision-making. Some decisions are very difficult to take; for example, whether to have a mastectomy or whether to give up alcohol or cigarettes. We need to allow time, to acknowledge that failures are allowed, and to plan with the patient suitable strategies for trying again. Most people will need support while taking a major decision, and while we cannot take the decision for them, we can provide some continuity of support.

As a result of your health promotion activities, patients should end up with more confidence, more autonomy and more choice. They should feel happy with their own decisions, rather than feeling that they have been pressurised into something they are not sure about, as can sometimes happen. Successful health promotion strengthens and enhances people and does not undermine them.

AM I A GOOD ROLE MODEL?

Finally, we will explore a dilemma which is faced by many nurses: how healthy do we have to be to qualify as a good health promoter? This is a worry which often stops us from attempting any health promotion as we feel that we are in no position to talk. The medical profession in general and nurses in particular are a pretty unhealthy bunch! We are usually over-stressed and tired. Each year approximately 764,000 working days are lost in the NHS because of back pain among nurses[6], although even more recent estimates[7] put the figure at 1.3 million days a year. In America it has been found that the psychiatrist is now more likely to commit suicide than his patients. Stress management — our own and that of our patients — is explored in *M3: Managing Stress*.

The most effective health promoters are nurses who are also aware of what makes them healthy, and so the first place to start is, of course, with yourself. Nobody expects you to be a paragon of virtue, or an Olympic athlete, but you will be much more credible to your patients if you appear to be attempting sensitively to practise what you preach.

Don't let feeling unhealthy prevent you from attempting health promotion with your patients; you could always plan a programme for both you and them!

FOCUS

Choose one of the health promotion opportunities you identified from your practice in the Focus for *P7(i): Health promotion: A question of choice.* Decide what you need to know to be better informed on the subject, then investigate the literature and write a report on the sources you will use.

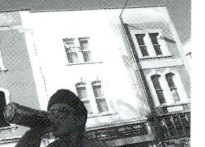

REFERENCES

1   Boore, J. *Prescription for Recovery.* London: RCN, 1978.
2   Hayward, J. *Information — A prescription against pain.* London: RCN, 1975.
3   Blennow, M., Granstrom, M., Jaatma, E., Olin, P. Primary immunisation of infants with an acellular pertussis vaccine in a double blind randomised clinical trial. *Pediatrics* 1979; **82**: 3, 293–299.
4   Tizard, B., Hughes, M. *Young Children Learning.* London: Fontana, 1984.
5   McKeown, T. *The Role of Medicine: Dream, mirage or nemesis?* London: Nuffield Provincial Hospitals Trust, 1976.
6   Watterson, A. Occupational health and illness: the politics of hazard education. In: Rodmell, S., Watt. A. (eds.) *The Politics of Health Education: Raising the issues.* London: Routledge and Kegan Paul, 1986.
7   *Nursing Times.* The hidden scandal. *Nursing Times* 1992; **88**: 41, 25–26.

FURTHER READING

•   Department of Health. *The Health of the Nation: A strategy for health in England.* London: HMSO, 1992.
•   Ewles, L., Simnett, I. *Promoting Health: A practical guide.* London: Scutari Press, 1992.
•   LeTouze, S., Calnan, M. Health promotion in general practice: The views of staff. *Nursing Times* 1996; **92**: 1: 32–33.
•   Tannahill, A. Health education and health promotion planning for the 1990s. *Health Education Journal* 1990; 49:194–198.
•   Whitehead, M., Tones, B. *Avoiding the Pitfalls.* London: Health Education Authority, 1991.

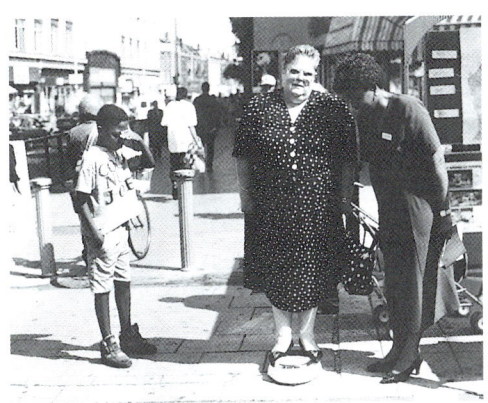 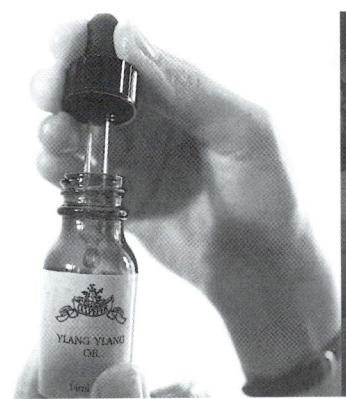 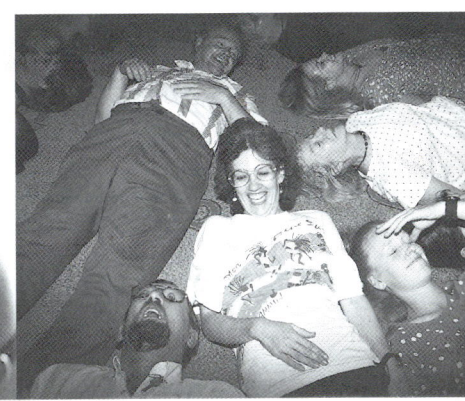

Planning a health promotion programme

Notes

In this final Part of *P7: Health Promotion*, you take a step-by-step look at how to plan an effective programme to promote the health of your patients.

The stages you will work through are:

- Assessment
- Goal-setting
- Formation
- Implementation
- Evaluation.

WORK PLANNER

For this Part you are asked to select a patient or group of patients for whom a health promotion programme is to be designed. In selecting such a group, you should carefully consider any ethical or organisational problems which might arise in using a patient group as 'guinea pigs' in this way, and clear your choice with the primary nurse, or whoever else is responsible for the patients' care. If there is any doubt as to whether or not you should use a group of patients, choose instead some other individuals you know, perhaps from among family or friends, and make sure you ask their permission before any discussion with them. You may find it helpful to refer to *P6: Facilitating Learning* when considering what sort of health promotion you are going to devise.

Activity 6 asks you to visit your local health promotion unit again, so you should schedule time to do this and make any necessary arrangements.

Remember, you can always contact your tutor/counsellor if you come up against a problem which you cannot solve yourself.

The unit *Healthcare in Professional Practice* in the Emap Healthcare Open Learning BSc (Hons) Professional Practice in Health Care has information on planning and health promotion in Section 5, 'Health promotion in practice'. (See the Introduction to this book, page 3, for details on how to obtain a copy.)

PLANNING FOR CHANGE

As explored in *P7(i): Health promotion: a question of choice?* and *P7(ii): Issues and dilemmas*, health promotion can be an integral part of our everyday work as we chat and talk to our patients. In providing them with accurate information about their health and behaviour as a matter of routine we can increase their choices about the future.

181

However, to achieve a major behaviour change, such as giving up smoking or reducing stress, we need a planned programme of health promotion, and this is the focus of our work here.

Many of the health-related behaviours which could increase our patients' chances of incurring serious illness are deeply enmeshed in their life-styles and cultures. To change or modify them requires tremendous effort on their part and a great deal of support from us. An essential point to remember is that our role is to *assist* with change, and not to *insist* on it.

We will break our planning down into five stages, although in practice you will probably find that they are all going on together, rather than taking place in a set order. However, it makes our job of discussing them easier if we take them in sequence, a sequence which you will no doubt recognise as the nursing process:

- **Assessment** of clients' health promotion needs

- **Setting goals** which are realistic and achievable

- **Deciding** on the form the programme should take

- **Implementing** the programme with clients

- **Evaluating** progress.

This last stage can lead to:

- **Reassessment** of the programme.

Let's look at each of these in more depth.

ASSESSMENT: THE ART OF THE POSSIBLE

Your first task in planning a programme of health promotion is to come to some sort of understanding with your patient, or patient's carer about the nature of the change he or she would like to embark upon.

Changing an aspect of a person's life-style is a difficult challenge for anyone, but in the case of health it may be the only option left. For example, patients who have just been diagnosed as having diabetes, or who have had a major heart attack, may have no choice but to alter radically many aspects of their lives. Under these circumstances, your role as a health promoter is to help these patients understand as much as possible about their condition, and the implications of *not* making changes, as well as of making them.

For other patients or clients, the achievement of better health may be a longer-term, less clearly defined issue, or one which can be achieved only over a longer period. For these patients, the motivation to change may come from a wish to feel better about themselves, to exert some control over their lives and their health.

ACTIVITY 1
knowledge base
For your selected group of patients or single patient (see Work Planner), briefly outline their major health promotion needs. Are these needs immediate or long-term?

FEEDBACK

The needs you identified in Activity 1 will probably have been those which you would like your patients to achieve in an ideal world. Your needs assessment should also take into account the factors which are acting against your clients changing their behaviour.

Making a full assessment of your clients' needs is an exercise in two of the communication skills discussed in *P6(i): Learning and communication* (listening and asking questions). The objective assessment you made in Activity 1 above must be tempered by an understanding of your clients' view of themselves and their views on health and illness. Discussions in *P1: Health and Illness; P2: Human Biography* and *P3: Human Environment* provided you with a basis for a realistic assessment of your patients' needs.

Your assessment should also consider factors relating to patients' current situations — their reactions to their present condition, their emotional needs, their position and role in the outside world, what support they can rely on from family and friends, and so on.

ACTIVITY 2
action
Now make a note of the things you want to find out about during informal contact with your selected patients; things that will help you to make a realistic assessment of their health promotion needs. Use the experience you gained in working through the previous Sections mentioned above to decide how you are going to approach this.

Your assessment should, in the end, provide you with an understanding of *what is possible* in the circumstances of each individual client.

SETTING GOALS: CHANGE IS POSSIBLE

Sometimes the possibility of change in our patients (or indeed in ourselves) seems an enormous challenge, but it is possible, and much easier once you get over the attitude that it is difficult. Our failures tend to stick in the mind much longer than our successes. We remember the broken New Year's resolutions and the abandoned diets rather than the achievement of what must have seemed like impossible tasks, such as riding a bicycle or driving a car, overcoming a fear of water or the dentist, or the unpleasant smell of hospitals.

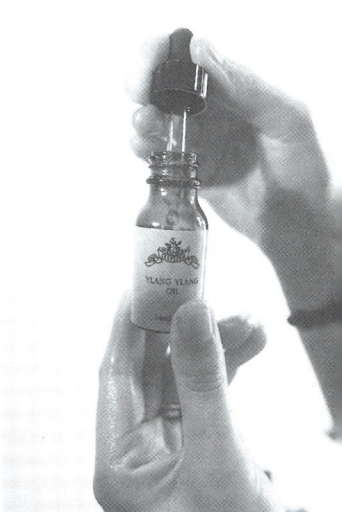

ACTIVITY 3
diary
Can you recall an occasion when you failed to keep a New Year's resolution about health? On reflection, why do you think you failed?

FEEDBACK

As you will no doubt be only too aware, there are many ways in which, even with the best intentions, we can fail in endeavours such as these. Perhaps you set yourself a very difficult target in the first place. Perhaps you tried to achieve something which was really a long-term goal in too short a period. Alternatively, your target may have been too poorly defined to be achievable — 'get thinner', 'eat less', 'cut down' ...
Would you have found it easier if you had set specific goals, such as 'cutting down to two bars of chocolate a week'? (you can plan to cut down to zero when you have achieved this).

ACTIVITY 4
diary
Identify either an aspect of your personality, or a health-related behaviour, that you would *really* like to change in yourself. It might be losing weight or taking more exercise, or something like being less critical or more organised.
Now try to specify *exactly* what it is you are going to change, and by when you intend that the change will be made. Make sure that your goal is realistic, and that you feel you would be able to achieve it.

FEEDBACK

We hope that this Activity has persuaded you of the need for clear thinking and straightforward honesty with yourself when setting goals. You might find it interesting to look back over your answers to Activity 4 and reflect on the process you went through; that is, how you decided what was realistic and achievable.

Goal-setting with your patients requires that you get them to go through a similar process; that is, that they set their own goals. As you may have discovered from your own experience of goal-setting, many people need guidance and support during this exercise. So you will now be in a position to guide your clients in setting their own health goals, having set the same goals for yourself.

ACTIVITY 5
action
Drawing on the information and experience you have gained from Activity 2, spend some time with the person you chose at the beginning of this Part (or one person from a group of patients) to set a clear, measurable goal which you both agree can be assessed.

EXAMPLES

You can also encourage your clients to draw on many other sources of support in setting goals. You might bring in other members of the healthcare team, or local branches of support groups. It might be possible to form groups of clients with similar conditions (for example, postnatal groups) or you might suggest the clients contact local support groups themselves (for example, the National Childbirth Trust, Weight Watchers).

The choices your clients make may well reflect a compromise between their needs and their existing life-styles. Part of the support you provide will be to encourage them to think through the implications of any changes they make. By doing this, their goals will seem more realistic, and therefore more achievable.

WHAT SHOULD GO INTO THE PROGRAMME?

Contrary to what many people believe, changing behaviour is not usually about will-power, or having strength of mind. Claxton[1] explains that what actually happens is that the mind goes through a subconscious decision-making process, weighing up all the pros and cons of changing, and the option that comes out best overall is what is actually done.

So we first need to inform our patients about their options, and then help them to analyse this information and support them as they decide what to do.

Methods of Providing Information

Providing information is one of the issues considered in *P7(ii): Issues and dilemmas* — the dilemma many nurses face about their own lack of information, and their inability to convey this information to others. We hope that your work for the Focus in P7: (ii) will have boosted your confidence in your own information base, and provided you with a system you can use when you next need to find out more.

You can add to this by investigating what health promotion materials might already be available and deciding whether or not they are appropriate to your own clients' needs, and how you might use them with the particular group of clients you have identified.

A one-to-one situation, such as a health visitor and mother, or a district nurse and a carer, will often be the most successful way of getting information across. Small groups, such as smoking-cessation groups or antenatal classes, are more effective when a certain amount of mutual support is important.

ACTIVITY 6
action
Visit your local health promotion unit, and find out what information it has on a subject relevant to your patient or group of patients. Bear in mind the goal you helped to set in Activity 5. Evaluate how useful you think this information would be by considering the following questions:
• Is it presented in an easily-followed format?
• Is the language easy to understand for all members of your client group? Is it produced in any language other than English?
• Could you easily adapt the material for any clients for whom it is not suitable in its present form?
• Are there any alternative sources, such as video, which might prove more effective?

You may also have come across some of the major media campaigns (AIDS, for example, or seat-belt legislation). These have had a very high profile and, in terms of the numbers of people reached, are easily the cheapest form of health promotion. However, it is less easy to determine their effect on individuals.

ACTIVITY 7
action
While you are at your health promotion unit, find out if any health promotion initiatives have been taken on a local basis. If not, has the unit identified any health problems which are particularly prevalent in your area?

You might also find it useful to investigate what is produced by any support groups working in your area.

ACTIVITY 8
action
Find out what health promotion information is available from any support groups working in the area in which you are interested. Compare this information with what you already have. Is it more/less suitable for your client group? Is it easy for clients to get hold of this information?

Now you are in a position to provide your patients with a wide range of information, either based on your own knowledge, or based on information supplied by other sources. The second part of the answer to the question 'What should go into the programme' focuses on how you can help your patients to use this information — in other words, how they are going to bring about the changes we have agreed are desirable.

IMPLEMENTING THE PROGRAMME

In general, methods which are active and enjoyable are more likely to be effective, where the emphasis is on supporting the patients' strengths, raising their confidence and self-esteem, rather than pointing out their faults, and making them feel guilty about their health-related behaviour.

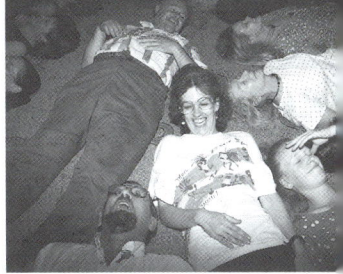

Change can be threatening because it challenges a person's beliefs about the sort of person he or she is. These beliefs may in fact be obsolete ones, left over from childhood and usually grounded in the need for acceptance and the fear of rejection. When threatened, the person may become rigid, dogmatic, inflexible, and therefore unreceptive to change.

Two Different Approaches to Change

Below, we consider briefly two approaches to the psychology of change. You will have to decide whether one or the other (or maybe neither) is most appropriate to any one client.

In the first approach, the clients work on the assumption that they are going to change, and prepare themselves mentally for being different people. They first need to have a clear picture of what they will be like when they have changed — then they have to behave as if they were already the people they would like to be. By doing this, they can identify and understand any problems in advance, and make suitable preparations to overcome them should they arise[2].

The second approach is a more practical one[3]: clients must consider three factors before they make changes. First, they need to be clear about their goal; that is, the task or job, or behaviour they need to change. Then they have to make an action plan, breaking down into small steps (or sub-goals) the stages of change. Finally, they need to take into consideration the emotions aroused and the people involved.

ACTIVITY 9
action
Turn again to Activity 4
and the change you would
like to make in yourself.
Choose one of the above
approaches and apply it.
Reflect on whether or
not it worked, and
why.

Deciding which of these approaches is best for each individual client is by no means easy. You may find that you 'waste time' by trying one approach which does not achieve very much. However, this is not wasted time — all the time you are learning more about your clients' needs, and providing them with feedback — and you will eventually find the best approach for each individual.

EVALUATION: HOW DID WE DO?

Sometimes you will be able to make a clear judgement about how successful a programme of health promotion has been. Your clients will give up smoking, learn to plan their time to include more relaxation, or whatever. But most of the time we have to face the fact that it isn't usually as easy as that, and that we have to evaluate not only how well we are doing, but more often the reasons why we aren't achieving as much with our clients as we would like. As explained in *P7(i): Health Promotion: A question of choice?*, however hard we try, there are other forces at work besides ourselves which are influencing our patients' health-related behaviour.

So what criteria can we use to judge how effective our programme of health promotion has been? The following list of questions provides a useful checklist[4].

- Was enough time spent in identifying the key characteristics of the person, setting a baseline and assessing the problem?

- Were the goals specific enough?

- Has the person 'bitten off more than he/she can chew'?

- Were the targets really mutually agreed or were they imposed by the helper?

- Were other people unhelpful?

- What other external pressures (time, unforeseen crises, and so on) hindered the outcome? What has been learnt from this?

- Have all the sources of support available to the person been fully exploited?

Answers to these questions can be used as the basis of a further assessment of the client's needs, and as the start of a further programme of health promotion if necessary.

A SUCCESSFUL PROGRAMME

For a successful planned programme following the stages we have discussed above, you will need to review your knowledge base and be sure you are up to date. Remember that your health promotion mentor is someone who can guide you to the latest reports and so save you considerable time.

You will need the best of communication skills, both with your clients and with your colleagues, who will need to be kept informed of what you are doing, so they can support your initiative.

FOCUS

Choose one of the following topics, or another which is relevant to your area of practice. Complete each stage of a health promotion programme, either for yourself, a friend or relative, or a patient:

- Smoking cessation

- Relaxation techniques

- Changing to a healthier diet

- Taking more exercise.

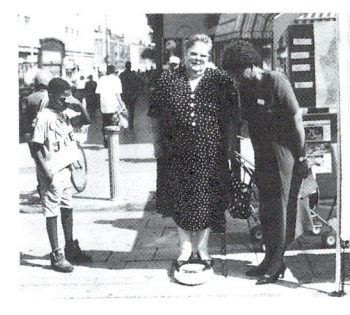

REFERENCES

1   Claxton, G. Beliefs and behaviour: Why is it so hard to change? *Nursing* 1987; **3**: 19, 670–73.

2   Bannister, D., Fransella, F. *Inquiring Man: The theory of personal constructs.* Harmondsworth: Penguin Books, 1971.

3   Handy, C. *Managing Organisations.* Harmondsworth: Penguin Books, 1985.

4   English National Board. *Health Promotion in Primary Healthcare. An open learning package for practice nurses.* London: ENB, 1989.

FURTHER READING

- Ewles, L., Simnett, I. *Promoting Health: A practical guide.* London: Scutari Press, 1992.

- Hall, C. *Advertising Emergency Contraception.* Rotherham: Rotherham Health Authority, 1995.

- Hall, C., Milner, P. Advertising emergency contraception using local radio: An evaluation. *Health Education Journal* 1996; **55**: 165–174.

- Kennedy, A. *Practising Health for All in a Glasgow Housing Scheme – The Drumchapel Healthy Cities Project 1990–1992.* Drumchapel: Drumchapel Community Health Project, 1994.

- Shepherd, J. The West Scotland Coronary Prevention Study: A trial of cholesterol reduction in Scottish men. *American Journal of Cardiology* 1995; **76**: 9, 1130–1170.

- Ahmad, W. I. U. (ed). *Race and Health in Contemporary Britain.* Buckingham: Open University Press, 1993.

- Dines, A., Cribb, A. (eds). *Health Promotion: Concepts and practice.* Oxford: Blackwell Science Ltd, 1993.

- Robinson, S., Hill, Y. The health promoting nurse. *Journal of Clinical Nursing* 1998; **7**: 3, 232–238.

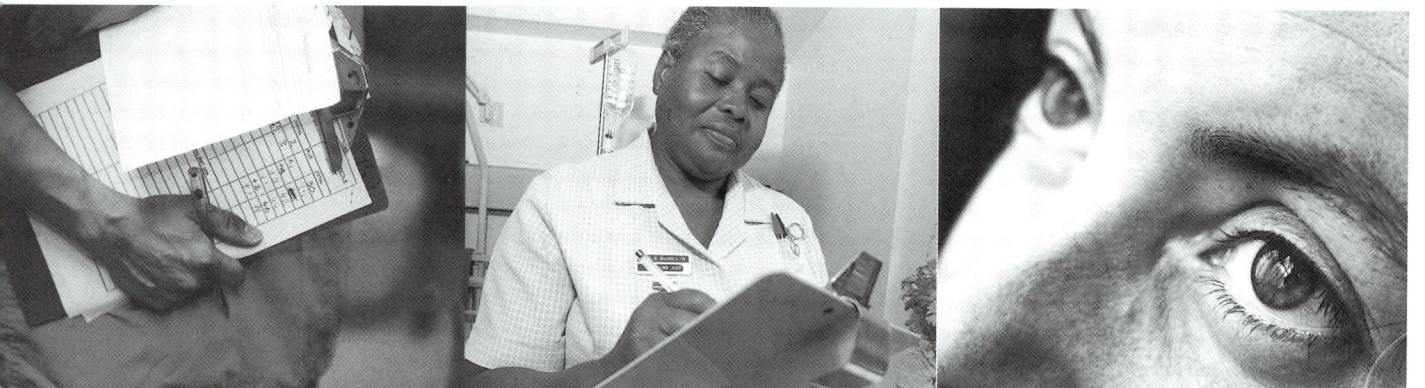

Ways of seeing

In order to decide how valuable a piece of research is to your practice, you need to understand how the researcher was thinking when he or she planned and carried out the research. This will give you a basis for understanding and evaluating the results of the research. In the three Parts of this Section, you will explore the different views which researchers can have of their subject matter, and examine how their choice of approach can influence the methods they use to carry out research.

In this Part you will learn about:

- Positivism — an approach in which the researcher is detached from the subject

- Interpretivism — an approach in which the researcher gets involved with the subject

- The difference between methods and methodology.

You will also look at:

- Why one approach is more suitable in some circumstances than in others

- The problems of categorising, that is, giving labels to people with different conditions

- Which methods are appropriate for a researcher to use.

WORK PLANNER

Activity 5 and the Focus ask you to refer back to the two research reports you used in *R2(iii): Reading research reports*. You will find it helpful to have these to hand as you work through this Part of the programme.

A QUESTION OF STRATEGY

At the end of *R2(iii): Focusing on Research Knowledge* we began to look at how to read research reports. We explored the questions that we can ask about any research report to help us understand how and why the research was carried out, and what the results were.

One of these questions was: 'What is the overall strategy?', that is, what general approach did the researcher take?

Here we investigate some of the different ways that researchers can approach their work. Understanding these differences is important in reading research because the overall approach usually influences the results of that research. This in turn affects the way we interpret the value of the research to us as practitioners. You will come across the terms 'quantitative' and 'qualitative'.

'Quantitative research is, as the term suggests, concerned with the collection and analysis of data in numeric form. It tends to emphasise relatively large-scale and representative sets of data, and is often, falsely in our view, presented or perceived as being about the gathering of 'facts'. Qualitative research, on the other hand, is concerned with collecting and analysing information in as many forms, chiefly non-numeric, as possible. It tends to focus on exploring, in as much detail as possible, smaller numbers of instances or examples which are seen as being interesting or illuminating, and aims to achieve "depth" rather than "breadth" '[1].

We will discuss quantitative and qualitative data collection in *R3(iii) The view from within: ethnography and phenomenology*. However, it is important to know that often these terms will be used to identify the differences in approach.

The differences we explore now are concerned with the way researchers view the subject they are researching.

ACTIVITY 1
knowledge base
Consider the following two studies of aspects of wound care.
Identify the main differences in the way the researchers approached their subject.
Study 1
This study examined techniques for cleaning wounds, and found that swabbing towards the wound encouraged bacteria to enter the wound and increase infection, while swabbing away from the wound discouraged infection. The results of the study depended on bacteria counts from wound swabs.
Study 2
This study investigated the experience of patients who were having wounds cleaned. The results showed that, for the majority of the sample, the experience was difficult and distressing. The results of the study were generated by lengthy interviews with patients who were having wounds dressed.

FEEDBACK

The two studies obviously look at two different aspects of wound care, but more than that, they use two different viewpoints. These two viewpoints are sometimes called *the view from above* and *the view from within*.

Study 1 is an example of the view from above. The researcher 'looks down' on what is going on, in a detached way. She assumes that she can understand what is going on without getting involved, and without communicating with the people, things or events she is studying. The 'connection' between the researcher and her subject is one-way.

Study 2 is an example of the view from within. In this case, the researcher tries to 'get inside' what is happening, and see the situation from the point of view of the participants. The connection here is two-way. The researcher recognises that there is a connection between herself and the subject, but she also recognises that the subject is the one who really knows what is going on.

The two approaches determine not only how the research is carried out, but also the way the results are analysed and presented. In the first study, the researcher could analyse her results on the basis of definitions (for example, 'increased infection') which she could make and we could all understand and share.

In the second study the situation is more complex. The researcher was trying to find out what the people concerned thought about the situation. She didn't make any assumptions based on her own understanding of what was going on, but asked the people to describe the situation in their own words, and accepted that what they had to say was important.

TWO DIFFERENT APPROACHES

These two approaches reflect two different 'ways of seeing' which have been used to study many different aspects of our society. These two important intellectual traditions have been given a number of different names, but here we will use the terms *positivism* and *interpretivism* for the two approaches we have just described.

Notes

- Positivism — the view from above

- Interpretivism — the view from within.

These terms reflect two fundamentally different attitudes to 'the way things are', and philosophers have devoted much time to discussing their relative merits. We need to understand them because, as we saw above, they represent a different view of the researcher and her role in research.

Positivism

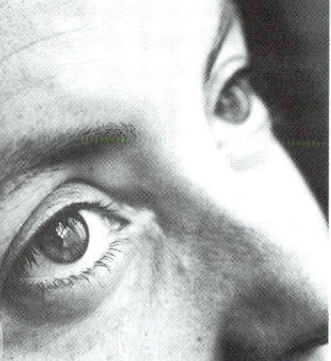

Positivists believe that people, things and processes exist independently of anyone trying to analyse them, and are governed by laws — what we might call the 'laws of nature'. The role of the researcher is to observe, and if necessary take things to bits, or test them to see how they really work, and what laws are operating. This 'way of seeing' has its origins in the 17th century, and evolved as people became more and more interested in explaining what they saw in the natural world around them.

Interpretivism is a tradition which has developed this century. As more and more of the physical and natural world was explained and understood by the scientists of the 19th century, others became more interested in explaining the *social* world — how societies are created and sustained. Interpretivists argue that 'social reality' is constructed not by a series of laws, but by the way individuals interact with each other.

Interpretivism

EXAMPLE

Interpretivists would suggest that nursing doesn't just exist 'out there' somewhere, waiting for people to become nurses, but that nursing is created by people interacting as nurses, doctors, patients, and so on, in particular ways. So there are no 'laws' to be discovered, only the different ways in which people understand and create the world.

Interpretivism has three main approaches:

- Phenomenology

- Ethnography

- Grounded theory.

Phenomenology investigates consciousness as experienced by the subject, the focus being the individual's interpretation of an experience.

Ethnography studies individual or group behaviour in their cultural or social environments. Phenomenology and ethnography are discussed in more detail in *R3(iii): The view from within: ethnography and phenomenology.*

Grounded theory is the generation of theories inductively, allowing the theory to come from the phenomena being studied. (Material in this Example is adapted from Parahoo[2].)

You may find these concepts difficult at the moment. But you will find as you carry on reading research material that you begin to see for yourself the very different approaches of viewing the world from above and viewing it from within. The terms positivism and interpretivism are just labels for concepts, but, like the terms 'qualitative' and 'quantitative' you do need to know them because many researchers identify their approaches using these terms.

We have, then, two very different traditions of thought which underpin much of the research we use in nursing. How do they compare?

WHICH APPROACH IS BETTER?

The use of the positivist approach in research led to an enormous increase in the understanding of events and processes in the natural world. For example, almost all of our knowledge of human physiology and pathology was developed in this way.

Because of this, researchers adopted the same approach when they began to study society in the late 19th century. However, people are not the same as physical objects, or organs of the body, and it became clear that studying the whole person and the way he or she behaved required a different approach to studying the liver or the spleen. This was even more the case when it came to studying a social group, such as nurses, or a *social process*, such as nursing.

In the following Activity we explore this further by trying to establish *why* studying social processes is different from studying physical processes. In both scenarios below, the researcher is adopting a positivist (view from above) approach.

ACTIVITY 2
knowledge base
Read both the scenarios which follow, then make some notes for each on any problems you can identify in the approach the researcher is using.
Example 1
A researcher is observing your conversation with a patient. Without discussing it with you, she categorises the interaction as 'aggressive', and suggests that your aggressive behaviour is due to the fact that your mother went out to work when you were very young.
Example 2
A researcher is studying sleep problems caused by admission to hospital. She asks you to identify which patients in your ward have sleep problems.

FEEDBACK

In both these cases, the researcher is creating problems for herself by trying to explain human behaviour in terms of a pre-determined set of ideas on how and why people behave the way they do.

In Example 1, you may have thought you were being very reasonable under difficult circumstances, or your behaviour might have been part of a long-standing joke between yourself and the patient. The researcher did not try to find out the reasons for your behaviour, but put her own interpretation on things.

Your account, at first hand, is known as a *first order* account, or *construct*. The researcher's interpretation is known as a *second order construct*. In research into the physical world, we can safely assume that the things we are researching, such as bacteria, trees or rocks, do not have first order constructs of themselves to influence the behaviour we are studying. However, in studying people or social processes, the views and opinions of the people involved are part of their behaviour, and we need to understand these in order to understand that behaviour.

In Example 2, there may be a similar problem, but there are now three possible views of the same situation. There is the patient's view, the nurse's view and the researcher's view of what might constitute a 'sleep problem'. This is by no means a simple matter, as a literature review on sleep problems will reveal[3].

MAKING CATEGORIES AND GIVING LABELS

In both our examples above, we have seen problems of *categorisation* and *interpretation*. In earlier Sections, we discussed some of the dangers of 'labelling' people, and then acting on our perceptions of what those labels mean (*P2: Human Biography, P5: Client Assessment*). Labelling can create even more problems when it comes to research.

Positivists will make consistent and identifiable categories on which they base their interpretation of their research findings. This is easy enough when studying bacteria, for example, but the above Activity shows that it is not so easy when it comes to studying social behaviour. The following extract illustrates this point further.

Austin et al.[4] describe a study comparing academic achievement between children with epilepsy and those with asthma to identify child perception, school adaptive functioning, and condition severity factors related to academic achievement 'Children with epilepsy had significantly lower achievement scores than children with asthma. Boys with severe epilepsy were most at risk for under-achievement. Factors related to poor academic achievement in both samples were: high condition severity, negative attitudes, and lower school adaptive functioning scores. Less variance was accounted for in the model for epilepsy ... than for asthma. Boys with seizure severity were most at risk for achievement-related problems'.

The extract describes how putting human behaviour into certain categories (in this case 'epilepsy and asthma') can influence the way we interpret that behaviour, that is, low academic achievers.

ACTIVITY 3
diary
Think of at least two examples of categories (either disease categories or work categories) which are central to your own role as a nurse. Reflect on where those categories came from (that is, who 'agrees' that they are a category?). In whose interests were these categories created?

FEEDBACK

All disease categories are *socially constructed*, that is, created by particular groups in society for the purpose of giving labels to people with different conditions.

These categories are created mainly for the convenience of other people, rather than for the benefit of the person wearing the label.

The Dangers of Labelling

Healthcare professionals, educationists and welfare officers may find it useful if someone has been labelled as having a 'learning disability'. They will all have an understanding of what the label means, making it easier for them to deal with the person wearing the label. The danger is that the label may not be a completely accurate representation of the individual.

Labelling people in this way can also create problems if our knowledge about the condition they are labelled with changes. There are examples from the history of medicine of disease categories which at one time seemed very 'concrete', but which have been largely or completely abandoned as knowledge and understanding of the condition have changed.

EXAMPLES

Hysteria was once widely used as a diagnosis[5], and miners' nystagmus was a well-documented syndrome in the 19th century[6], but neither is used much to describe clients' conditions nowadays.

So to answer the question 'which approach is better — positivism or interpretivism?' we can say that the positivist framework, in which we view our subject from above, and categorise its behaviour in terms of widely agreed laws, is more suitable for some types of subject matter than others. It is also more appropriate for seeking out some types of information than others.

Notes

ACTIVITY 4
knowledge base
Take two aspects of patient care; how much patients weigh and the pain they are experiencing. If you were beginning some research on these aspects, which of the two approaches we have been looking at would you choose for each?

FEEDBACK

The positivist approach would be more appropriate for studying weight. There are agreed measures for weight which everyone uses and understands, so you would weigh your patients and analyse the findings. You would not need to get involved with the patients and ask questions such as: 'How much do you feel you weigh?'

However, this approach would not be suitable if you wanted to look at how people felt about their weight, nor for the amount of pain they are experiencing. There are no objective scales for measuring these aspects. The 'view from within' would seem to be the more useful approach here.

The simple examples which you looked at in the Activity 4 should help you to understand the two approaches we have been discussing.

METHODS AND METHODOLOGY

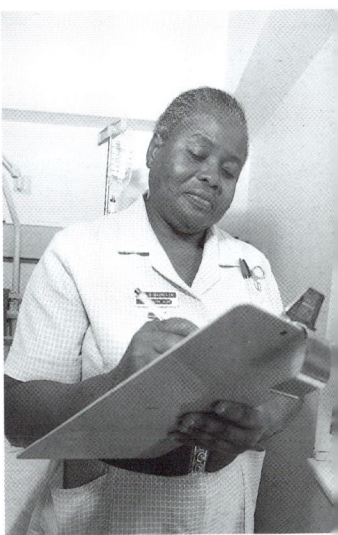

The choice of research approach is important because it determines many other things about how the research is carried out. It determines how the researcher sees her subject matter, how she believes it (or they) behaves, and therefore whether she thinks it is best studied by experiments and surveys, for example, or by actually becoming involved with the subject matter herself. This overall view of how the research will be done is known as its *methodology*.

Parts (ii) and (iii) of this Section on *Research Approaches*, explore the main research methodologies used in each of our two main research frameworks — positivism and interpretivism.

The choice of methodology in turn determines the choice of research *method*, that is, the specific research activities which are used to collect and analyse data. There are many different types of research method, and as you read more and more research, you will no doubt encounter most of them. Researchers can collect data using questionnaires and interviews, experiments or observation. They can also use secondary data (see *R2(iii): Reading research reports*) such as healthcare records and government statistics as the basis for analysis.

The following extract sets out the differences between method and methodology:

'Research methods are the tools and techniques used to carry out and analyse a piece of research: tools such as questionnaires and techniques such as interviewing. Research methodology, on the other hand, is the theoretical assumption upon which the choice of a particular research method is made. Methodology is a philosophical matter concerned with both theories of knowledge and, in the social sciences, theories about the nature of social reality and the relationship between human beings and society. So before we can decide how to find out about social life — that is, which methods to use — we have to work out how we know what we know and what it is we want to know about. Methodological issues crucially affect that decision[7].'

Notes

ACTIVITY 5
knowledge base
Read the extract on the previous page again, and identify two research methods mentioned. Use them to begin a collection of notes on research methods. You could keep a section of your diary for your notes, and add to them each time you meet a new research method. Alternatively, you could keep a section of your card index file for research methods, with a card for each method. Look back to your notes on the research articles you read in *R2(iii) Reading research reports*. Make a list of the research methods used, and add to your notes as many examples of other methods as you can.

FEEDBACK

The two methods mentioned in the extract are questionnaires and interviewing.

CAN WE SAY WHICH METHODS ARE BEST?

The whole range of research methods, including those outlined above, is available to any researcher, regardless of the approach that is adopted.

As we saw earlier, how researchers choose to collect their data depends on their view of how their subject matter behaves. In general, things which behave according to clearly defined and understood laws are best studied by experiment and survey, which can test their behaviour against precise criteria. This does not always mean 'things' rather than 'people' — a lot of market research, for example, uses survey methods to find out and categorise the views of different groups in society on very specific subjects.

On the other hand, researchers adopting the phenomenological approach are more likely to use interviews and observation, to 'get inside' the behaviour of their subjects, rather than to label it on the basis of judgements made by the researcher.

Just as we saw that one *approach* was not necessarily better than the other, only more or less appropriate to a particular situation, so no particular *method* is better than any other — it just depends how it is used.

In deciding which method to use, a researcher will consider three questions about the method and the data it produces:

- How *reliable* is it
- How *valid* is it
- How *representative* is it

} in the circumstances in which it is used?

These are also important questions for anyone evaluating a piece of research to ask, so we will now explore what these terms mean.

ACTIVITY 6
diary
The terms 'valid', 'reliable' and 'representative' are all words we use in everyday conversation. Write a brief note on your understanding of each.

FEEDBACK

These terms have a specialised meaning in research. Read the definitions below, and compare them with your everyday definitions.

'**Reliability** If a method of collecting evidence is reliable, it means that anybody else using this method, or the same person using it at another time, would come up with the same results. The research could be repeated, and the same results would be obtained.

Notes

'For example, an experiment in a chemistry lesson should always 'work'. It should always produce the result that is expected, whoever is doing it, at whatever time, provided that the proper procedures are followed.

'**Validity** Validity refers to the problem of whether the data collected are a true picture of what is being studied. Are they really evidence of what they claim to be evidence of? The problem arises particularly when the data collected seem to be a product of the research method used rather than of what is being studied.

'**Representativeness** This refers to the question of whether the group of people or the situation that we are studying are typical of others. If they are, then we can safely conclude that what is true of this group is also true of others ... If we do not know whether they are representative, then we cannot claim that our conclusions have any relevance to anybody else at all'[8].

These definitions represent an ideal world of research, where for every method we could answer 'yes' to each of the questions we asked above.

However, some research methods used in some circumstances are more reliable and representative than others; some may be more valid.

ACTIVITY 7
diary
Turn again to the two aspects of patient care you looked at in Activity 4 — the patient's weight and experience of pain. Which methods of research would you use if you were carrying out research into these areas? Choose methods for each which are likely to produce data which is reliable and valid.

FEEDBACK
Anyone carrying out research into weight would carry out a data-gathering exercise by weighing all the patients in the group. This would be reliable, as anyone else weighing the same group of patients correctly would get the same information. This is likely to be valid in that the actual weight of each person in the group could be said to be a true picture of what is being studied. How representative the method is would depend on the nature of the group, which we have not specified here.

Measuring pain levels would be done by interviews and observation. These would be reliable methods in as much as a patient would be likely to give the same reply to two different interviewers if his condition was the same. The validity of the interview method here would depend on the questions in the interview.

In *R3(ii): The view from above: experiments and surveys* we explore some of these issues further by looking in more detail at some of the research methodology and methods used by researchers who adopt the 'view from above', and in *R3(iii): The view from within: ethnography and phenomenology* we explore the methods and methodologies of those who adopt the 'view from within'.

FOCUS

Look back to the two research reports you studied in *R2(iii): Reading research reports* and identify:

- The approach — is the researcher taking a positivist or interpretive view?

- The methodology — what are the theoretical assumptions underlying the researcher's choice of methods?

- The methods — what techniques and/or tools is the researcher using?

Write three or four short paragraphs on each, explaining why you think the researcher chose these as the most appropriate for the particular subject that was being studied.

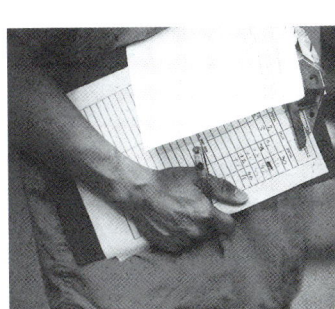

Notes   ## REFERENCES

1   Blaxter, L., Hughes, C., Tight, M. *How to Research*. Buckingham: Open University Press, 1996.
2   Parahoo, K. *Nursing Research. Principles, processes and issues*. London: Macmillan, 1997.
3   Closs, J. Assessment of sleep in hospital patients: A review of methods. *Journal of Advanced Nursing* 1988; **13**: 501–510.
4   Austin, J.K., Huberty, T.J, Huster, G.A., Dunn, D.W. Academic achievement in children with epilepsy. *Developmental Medicine and Child Neurology* 1998; **40**: 4, 248–255.
5   Open University. *Medical Knowledge: Doubt and certainty*. OU Course U205, Book 2, 1985.
6   Figlio, K. How does illness mediate social relations? Workman's compensation and medico-legal practices 1890–1940. In: Wright, P., Treacher, A. (eds.) *The Problems of Medical Knowledge*. Edinburgh: Edinburgh University Press, 1982.
7   Sidell, M. How do we know what we think we know? In: Brechin, A., Walmsley, J. (eds) *Making Connections*. London: Hodder & Stoughton, 1989.
8   McNeil, P. *Research Methods*. London: Tavistock, 1985.

FURTHER READING

•   Cormack, D.F.S. (ed) *The Research Process in Nursing* (3rd edn.). Oxford: Blackwell Science, 1996.
•   Roberts, H. (ed) *Doing Feminist Research*. London: Routledge, 1981.

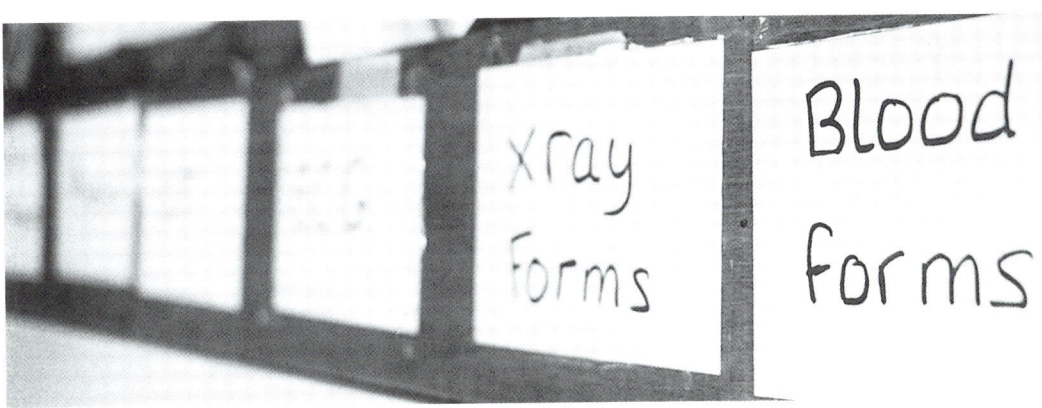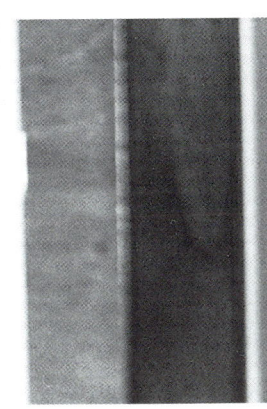

The view from above: experiments and surveys

What are the main methods of research used by researchers adopting the view from above, and what sorts of questions should we ask to determine how valuable such research is to us? In this Part you will be examining some of the research methods used within the positivist tradition. We begin by answering an important question: 'Why do I need to know about how research is done?'

We go on to help you understand:

- Researchers and the research process
- What a survey is
- How to evaluate experimental research
- The similarities and differences between experiments and surveys.

WORK PLANNER

Here and in *R3(iii): The view from within: ethnography and phenomenology* we look at some of the different research methods used. While you study these, try to arrange to spend as much time as possible in your college nursing library looking at a range of different research material on a subject that interests you, and familiarising yourself with the different methods used.

Activity 1 asks you to visit your college of nursing library and collect articles on a subject in which you are interested. You will need to refer to these articles during your work here.

WHY DO I NEED TO KNOW ABOUT HOW RESEARCH IS DONE?

Understanding some of the practical issues relating to research will help you to judge how relevant a particular piece of research is to your own area of work. Here and in Part (iii) *The view from within: ethnography and phenomenology* you will explore how these pitfalls, problems and pressures can influence the results of research. You will consider how you can apply the three criteria of quality discussed in *R3(i): Ways of seeing*: reliability, validity and representativeness.

Notes

We will concentrate on three major methodologies:

- Surveys
- Experiments
- Ethnography.

RESEARCHERS

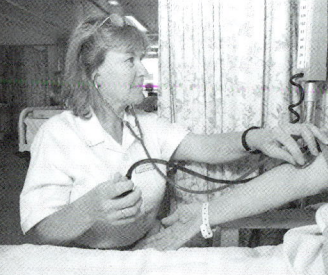

The first point to bear in mind when evaluating any research methodology is that research never takes place in an ideal world. No method or approach can give perfect results — each has its own particular strengths and drawbacks. What we have to do is to appreciate the limitations within which research takes place, and base our evaluation on a realistic view.

Researchers are not perfect people. Like most of us, researchers often find that the pressure to do things, or to produce something, is so great that they don't have as much time as they would like to think about doing research.

THE RESEARCH PROCESS

Although surveys and experiments may seem very different, both seek to explain the behaviour of people or things in relation to certain laws. This involves the researcher taking a view on what she thinks is likely to happen, and then producing the research to support or contradict this view.

The 'view' that the researcher has of the subject is therefore a key issue in determining the nature of the research. This view, or hypothesis, is a sort of hunch about the phenomenon being studied. The research process involves formulating a *hypothesis*, carrying out the research to obtain data relating to that hypothesis, and then analysing the data to determine whether or not the hypothesis was 'right'.

HYPOTHESIS ⟶ DATA COLLECTION ⟶ ANALYSIS

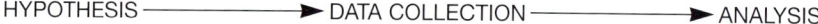

The analysis of data is carried out using a series of statistical laws known as probability. These statistics are used to indicate how far what happened was due to chance, and how far it can be explained by the researcher's hypothesis. Researchers are often reluctant to talk about 'cause and effect', but prefer to consider the degree to which two different events are related to one another. So, rather than say: 'This research *proves that* x was caused by y,' they would prefer to say 'This research *indicates that there is a close relationship between* the incidence of x and y'.

So what are the main characteristics of these two research methodologies?

SURVEYS

In the course of your reading, you are almost certain to have come across a number of surveys. They are probably the most common form of research in nursing, and they are also very widespread in everyday life (they are used in market research, for example).

FEEDBACK

If you are very canny, you will have chosen an article which started 'This survey ...'. But there are characteristics which will help you identify a piece of work as being a survey even if the researcher is less specific, or calls it something else.

In your answer to Activity 2, you may have said that surveys are characterised by the use of *questionnaires* or *structured interviews* to ask questions, or that *observers* note down details of events, such as numbers of particular types of vehicles passing a fixed spot. You may also have noted that surveys usually cover a sample of the total population they are trying to study.

What we have identified here are *methods* of collecting data. But there is more to defining a survey than that. Read the following definition of a survey:

'... any enquiry which collects pieces of information, by whatever method, over a range of different cases, and arranges the information about those cases as variables; variables therefore must have the property of providing one unique code for every case'[1].

ACTIVITY 3
diary
Read again the definition above of a survey. Underline what it says about *collecting* information/data, and write a brief comment on what is said.

FEEDBACK

By using the words 'by whatever method', the writer of the definition above says that how the information is collected is *not* an important characteristic of a survey.

ACTIVITY 4
diary
Now read the definition again and note down what it says about *analysing* the data.

FEEDBACK

The writer says that the data must be *arranged as variables*. Starting with the word 'variable', we are going to look at what is meant by this.

A variable is part of something which can be defined and examined in isolation from all other parts of the situation. In a traffic survey, the type of vehicle might be a variable, or the direction in which it is travelling. In a survey of people, their sex might be a variable, or their social class, or age, or attitude to old people, or use of learning materials.

Marsh[1] says that a variable 'must have the property of providing one unique code for every case'. This means that each item in the survey can belong to only one category of each variable.

EXAMPLE

In our traffic survey, a vehicle is *either* a lorry, or a car, or a bus, or some other type of vehicle. It cannot belong to more than one category. In our 'people' survey, the subject is either male or not male, social class 1 or another social class, and so on.

What about 'arranged'? In deciding which variables she is going to use, the researcher imposes a pattern on the data she is collecting. She will identify a *dependent* variable, which is the thing or group of things whose behaviour she wants to study, and one or more *independent* variables, which are the things that will influence the behaviour of the dependent variable.

EXAMPLE

We will illustrate this by returning to our traffic survey. The researcher might decide that she wants to know something about the types of vehicle which use a particular road junction at different times of day. The type of vehicle would be the dependent variable, and the time of day the independent variable. On the other hand, she might decide that the type of vehicle was not important to her survey — that some other factor, such as age, or country of origin was more important.

The survey researcher can choose her variables and allocate data to them in any way she sees fit. One major consideration will be the need to categorise *all* the items of data she collects — she can't throw items of data away just because they don't 'fit'.

So surveys are characterised by the type of data and what is done with the data, rather than by the method of collecting data. Our traffic researcher might sit on the same street corner, and count exactly the same vehicles, but arrange them in a different way depending on what was to be studied.

ACTIVITY 5
knowledge base
Look again at your example of a survey which you identified in Activity 2. Identify the dependent and independent variables. Now identify the process of arranging the data. Are you still satisfied that this is a survey? If not, choose another article and go on until you are fairly confident that you have found a survey.

Judging the Quality of Research Based on Surveys

One problem is *validity* — that is, are the data collected a true picture of what is being studied, or has the researcher 'arranged' the data to tell the story intended to be told at the beginning? Researchers can fall into this trap quite easily, not necessarily because they want to deceive, but because in attempting to establish some sort of order on the world they are studying, they can create a false picture of what is actually going on.

A second problem is *representativeness* — that is, are the data representative of other groups of people or things, or just of the group being studied? Can we *generalise* from the study to our own situation? Generalisability depends on the *population* being studied. The population is the whole group in which the researcher is interested.

ACTIVITY 6
knowledge base
Consider each of the research questions listed below[2].
Make a note of the population in each (it is not always explicitly stated). How does each population relate to your workplace?
Write short notes on whether the research into each question would be generalisable to your situation.
• What is the content of one-to-one (dyadic) nurse/patient verbal interactions in surgical wards? What are the dynamics of these situations and what verbal strategies are employed by nurses?
• What do hospital patients think about their stay in hospital following discharge?
• What is the utilisation of the prophylactic child health services currently available within the National Health Service for infants during the first 24 months of life?
• What are the demands of leg ulcer care on the National Health Service?

FEEDBACK

Being able to identify the population and decide how representative it is of other groups is an important step in evaluating research. Your answers to Activity 6 will obviously depend on your own area of work. For example, if you work in a surgical ward, there is a good chance that our first research question will produce some results which are generalisable to your own situation. However, you may work in another type of acute ward and decide that the findings have some relevance to your situation as well, or you may work somewhere where the first research question has no relevance to you at all.

You may find Parahoo's book, *Nursing Research: Principles, processes and issues*[3] useful as a framework for considering the questions listed in Activity 6.

We have now considered some of the broad issues relating to the value of survey-based research. There is a whole range of other issues which relate to some of the methods used, and you will be able to explore some of these by further reading as you encounter them.

EXPERIMENTS

You probably remember the general framework of experiments from your days in school science classes. As in surveys, experiments study the behaviour of different variables. The role of the researcher is to control the environment and change one variable in order to demonstrate the role of that variable.

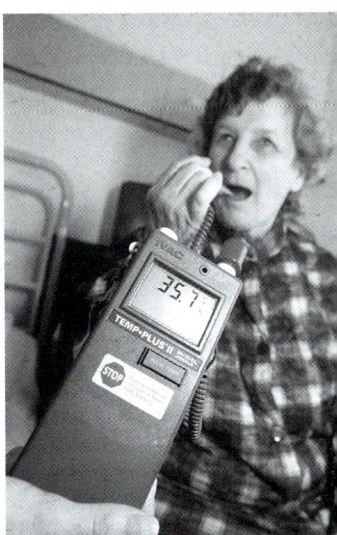

EXAMPLE

A group of bacteria could be sprayed with an antibiotic to see what happens. The bacteria are the dependent variable, and the antibiotic the independent variable. In such a case a second group of bacteria would be kept in identical circumstances, but not sprayed with an antibiotic.

The researcher would expect that the bacteria would be killed by the antibiotic, but would not know that they were not killed by some other factor, such as cold, unless other bacteria were kept in the same conditions. This second group is called a *control*.

As *R3(i): Ways of seeing* explained, experimental research is one of the major ways in which we understand the physical world. However, it can also be used to study the behaviour of social groups.

> **ACTIVITY 7**
> **knowledge base**
> Read the brief account below of experimental research, and the definition of an experiment. For each of the characteristics of experiments listed in extract 2, underline the part of the account in extract 1 which describes that characteristic.

Extract 1: '324 adults in hospital for a minimum of 2 days for non-cardiac surgery. Adults were included if they smoked and were ready to quit smoking ... 168 adults were randomly allocated to an intervention that was administered by a public health educator. The individualised programme lasted 30 – 60 minutes and included viewing a 10-minute video tape and counselling ... ; assessment of and countermeasures to barriers to quitting smoking; self-management techniques ...; assessment and referral for depression; and a 3-month prescription and instructions on the use of nicotine gum or patch; 5 follow-up calls were also made over 5 months. 156 patients were allocated to a control group and received a 10-minute counselling session on the risks of smoking and benefits of quitting. Outcome measures were self-reported and laboratory-confirmed quit rates using serum or saliva samples for continue testing'[4].

Extract 2: 'In a true experiment ..., the researcher:

1. Manipulates the experimental situation by systematically varying one or more variables ...

2. Introduces some control over the experimental situation by eliminating the influence of variables other than those manipulated by the experimenter ...

3. Randomly assigns people (or objects) to the different groups which take part in the experiment.'[5]

FEEDBACK

The research which was described in Extract 1 above is an example of a *randomised controlled clinical trial*.

The independent variable in this example was the individualised programme as it was given to an individual. The dependent variables which were observed for change were self-reports on quitting and laboratory-confirmed continue tests.

You may have found some difficulty finding evidence for the elimination of other variables. There was a second group to whom no individualised programme was given, which acted as a control. However, there is very little the researcher can do in such a situation to eliminate other variables, such as the influence of society in general on the people being studied. This is one of the major problems of taking the experimental method out of the laboratory.

The people were randomly allocated to different groups ('adults were randomly allocated ... to the individualised programme').

Experimental research which takes place outside the laboratory is known as *field research*, and the randomised controlled clinical trial is one variation of this.

ACTIVITY 8
action
Look through your selected research articles to find an account of an experiment. Again, use the definition of an experiment in Extract 2 above to check your decision. If you are not happy that your example is covered by this definition, find another example and try again.

Evaluating Experimental Research

We will now look at the factors which can influence the results of such research. The questions of validity and representativeness that we considered in relation to surveys are also relevant here. The choice of population to be studied, and the variables about which the data are arranged are just as important when reading experimental research.

When reading reports of experimental research on social groups, the question of *reliability* also arises. Laboratory research can control the environment fairly tightly, and the thing being studied (assuming that it is not human) does not have its own opinions to get in the way of research. Anyone doing the same experiment under identical conditions would be likely to get the same result. However, in experimental studies of groups of people, they usually know what is going on. This has been called the 'Hawthorne Effect'.

EXAMPLE

'In 1927, Professor Elton Mayo of Harvard University designed an experiment about the relationship between working conditions, workers' tiredness, and their productivity. He set up a test area in a factory making telephone relays, with five female volunteers who knew the experiment was taking place. Working conditions were matched with those in the main working area, and Mayo then varied such things as room temperature, humidity, hours of work, and rest breaks. Observation in the first few months showed that, almost regardless of what changes were made, output went up, even when conditions were apparently worsened.

Five hypotheses were suggested to explain this, and each was tested. The most convincing turned out to be that the girls were responding to being involved in the experiment, and were developing strong group loyalties and a wish to please the experimenters'[6].

ACTIVITY 9
knowledge base
Read the account above again. Think of some ways in which the Hawthorne Effect might have been avoided in this case, and make some notes about those aspects of the experiment which could have been conducted differently.

FEEDBACK

The 'girls' in the factory knew that an experiment was going on, and so altered their behaviour. How could this have been prevented, except by keeping them in ignorance about what was going on? If people did not know, they would not have altered their behaviour, but would it be ethical not to tell them?

SIMILARITIES AND DIFFERENCES BETWEEN EXPERIMENTS AND SURVEYS

We have explored two of the major research methodologies used within the positivist framework — surveys and experiments — and have identified some of the questions you should ask when evaluating such research. We want to end by considering what these methodologies have in common and how they differ.

Both formulate a hunch, or hypothesis, which they want to test. They then identify one or more dependent variables, and a series of independent variables. They will try to explain changes in the behaviour of the dependent variable by relating them to variations in the independent variable, and will use statistical tools known as probability to determine how closely one is related to the other.

Where they differ is in the structure of the process used to achieve this. In the experimental method, the structure is as follows:

Experiment

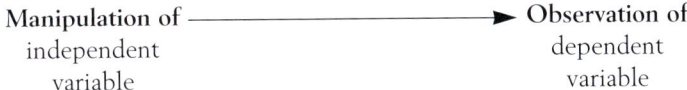

Manipulation of ——————————→ Observation of
independent   dependent
variable   variable

Experimenters 'do something to' their subjects (and usually 'do not do something to' a set of controls), and look to see what effect changing the independent variable has on the dependent variable. Within the limits defined by the laws of probability, experimenters can be sure that it is what they did to the independent variable that has produced any variance they observed in the dependent variable.

In a survey, it is not always so easy to manipulate the independent variable. Suppose the independent variable was 'social class'. How can you manipulate someone's social class? In this case, the researcher observes both the dependent variable and the independent variable, and tries to find a statistical relationship between them.

Survey

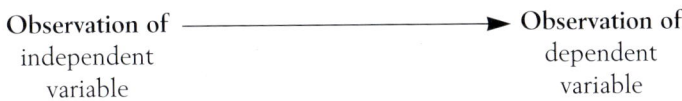

Observation of ——————————→ Observation of
independent   dependent
variable   variable

Interpreting the results of survey research carried out in this way can create yet another problem. The research might show that there is a statistical relationship between two variables — for example, sugar consumption and the incidence of cancer. As we said at the beginning of this Part, researchers are often reluctant to talk about cause and effect, and this example illustrates why. Can we assume from this that eating sugar causes cancer, or is there another factor that we haven't considered? For example, eating sugar damages your teeth, and bad teeth might cause cancer.

Notes

**ACTIVITY 10
knowledge base**
Suggest some other variables that might intervene between the eating of sugar and the incidence of cancer.

Both these approaches — survey and experiment —'take the world to pieces' in order to try to understand specific aspects of it. We have explored some of the issues which arise from this for our understanding of such research and its value to our practice. In *R3(iii): The view from within: ethnography and phenomenology* we explore a methodology which tries to preserve the 'wholeness' of the world it studies as much as possible, using the view from within.

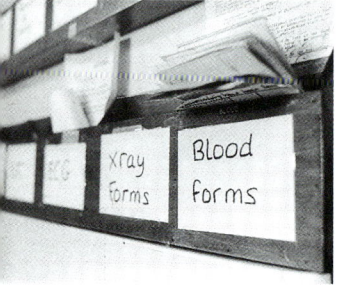

FOCUS

Take one example of a survey and one example of an experiment from your collection of articles. For each one, think about how the research could have been done using the 'view from within'. For example, if you look back at the experiment described in Extract 1 on page 201, the researcher would have had to work with counselling groups whichever approach was used, but the methods used to get information would have been different if the researcher was using the 'view from within'.

What do you think would have been gained in terms of understanding, and what lost, by this 'translation' of approaches?

REFERENCES

1   Marsh, C. Problems with surveys, method or epistemology? In: Bulmer, M. (ed) *Sociological Research Methods: An introduction.* (2nd edn.) London: Macmillan, 1984.

2   Macleod Clark, J., Hockey, L. *Further Research for Nursing.* Harrow: Scutari Press, 1989.

3   Parahoo, K, *Nursing Research. Principles, processes and issues.* London: Macmillan, 1997.

4   Simon, J.A., Solkowwittz, S.N., Carmody, T.P. et al. Smoking cessation after surgery: A randomised trial. *Evidence-Based Nursing* 1998; **1**: 2.

5   Distance Learning Centre. *The Experimental Perspective.* London: DLC Research Awareness Series, 1988.

6   McNeill, P. *Research Methods.* London: Tavistock Publications, 1985.

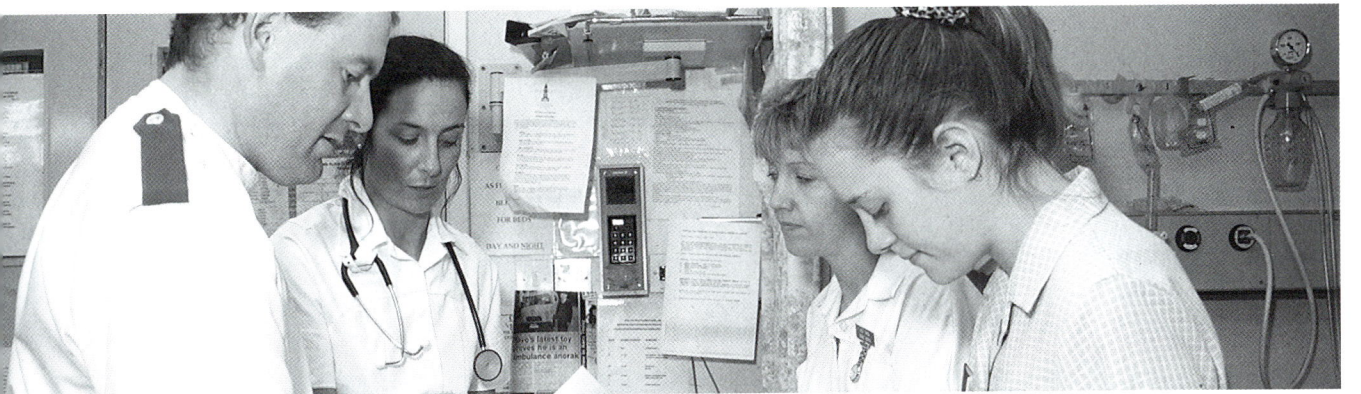

The view from within: ethnography and phenomenology

This Part looks at the methods used by researchers in the interpretive tradition to study their subject matter.

You will be:

- Considering the problems in interpreting phenomenological and ethnographical work
- Learning about three ethnographic and phenomenological research methods:
    - Observation
    - Unstructured interviews
    - Conversation analysis
- Considering the difference between qualitative and quantitative research.

Notes

WORK PLANNER

Activity 3 asks you to observe activities at your place of work as a 'stranger'. Read through the Activity in advance and seek any permission that might be necessary to do this.

Activity 7 asks you to obtain and use a small tape recorder to tape conversations between people you know well. Before you do this, make sure you have their permission to do so (although it might be wise to wait a while after asking so that the fact that they are being taped is not at the front of their minds).

GETTING THE INSIDE VIEW

The terms phenomenology and ethnography mean 'writing about a way of life'. They are the main research methodologies within the interpretivist framework — the view from within. They are probably the most accessible types of research for other people, because they are descriptive, and almost always a 'good read'.

Unlike the positivist researchers whose work is considered in *R3(ii): The view from above: experiments and surveys*, ethnographers and phenomenologists do not base their work on hunches or hypotheses. Rather, they seek to tell the whole story, with the expectation that ideas about why things are the way they are will emerge as a result of their work.

Ethnographers and phenomenologists do not believe that social life can be reduced to a series of variables; they believe that it needs to be dealt with *holistically*, that is, as a whole. So if, for example, a phenomenologist is basing an argument on a set of answers to a particular question, some of the actual answers to the question would be included to show that the explanation was grounded in 'reality'.

The following is an extract from an account of phenomenological work on student nurses' lived experiences of the sudden death of their patients:

'The researcher, Linda, asked an initial interview question: "Reflect on a specific experience of caring for a dying patient." Other questions would then be used to prompt where necessary.

Helen and Mary explain how they were not prepared for their patients' sudden deterioration.

'She was walking about, she got there. She was quite sort of bright. We got on really well. Then after my days off she was in bed. I was really shocked at the difference in her. She was hardly opening her eyes or anything. She was sleeping a lot of the time and she died a few days later.' (Helen)

'How did you feel about this?' (Linda)

'It was a shock. I liked her a lot. Yes, it was quite upsetting, because it was so sudden for me, but looking back the staff were quite aware of it.' (Helen)

Mary also came back from days off and found that her patient, unexpectedly to her, had deteriorated. She found that she felt angry and let down.

'I was really shocked at how she was. I did feel angry at this. I felt terrible afterward. I didn't realise at the time how seriously ill she was. I felt at times really angry because she seemed to give up. She just didn't seem to want to go on anymore and I couldn't understand her. I could understand her being depressed, but I couldn't understand why she didn't want to try. I didn't realise she was so ill. I'd seen other patients who looked unwell but they got better.' (Mary)

Mary's cultural background and upbringing strongly influenced her first experience of a patient dying. She admitted that she expected her patients to get better and was unprepared for the fact that some of them would die[1].

ACTIVITY 1
knowledge base
Can you identify any problems for the reader in interpreting the results of such research? Think about the three criteria — reliability, validity and representativeness.

FEEDBACK
Looking back to our three criteria we can see that this seems to provide a *valid* account of what the researcher observed. Her report indicates that *some* of the nurses she spoke to gave the replies indicated, and that the statements given by nurses experiencing similar situations supported each other.

However, because she has not reproduced all her data for the reader, she may be open to the charge that she has picked out only the parts of the database which support her argument.

We may also question how far the particular group the phenomenologist chose to study is *representative* of other similar groups: in our example above, how typical are the student nurses' experiences described here compared with those of nurses in general?

As explained in *R3(i): Ways of seeing*, reliability and representativeness are not always appropriate to the 'view from within'. Ethnographers and phenomenologists do not often claim to produce results which are generalisable to other situations.

ETHNOGRAPHIC RESEARCH METHODS

Ethnography differs from phenomenology in that it concentrates on the behaviour of individuals as opposed to the individual's interpretation of experience.

In the example above, we briefly considered one method commonly used by phenomenological researchers — asking questions. *R3(ii): The view from above: experiments and surveys* explained that asking questions was a common research method for researchers carrying out surveys. Shortly, we will be exploring ethnography and how the two methodologies, surveys and ethnography, differ. But first we want to explore some of the other research methods used by ethnographers:

- Observation

- Unstructured interviews

- Conversation analysis.

The ideal position for the ethnographer is to be immersed in the situation being studied, living within the group and observing the behaviour of its members without changing it. This method is derived from the 19th-century anthropologists who went out from the United States and Britain to study island societies in the Pacific. One of the most distinguished anthropologists offered this advice to researchers:

'The anthropologist must relinquish his comfortable position in the long chair on the verandah of the missionary compound, Government station, or planter's bungalow, where, armed with pencil and notebook and at times with whisky and soda, he has been accustomed to collect statements from informants, write down stories, and fill out sheets of paper with savage texts. He must go out into the villages, and see the natives at work in the gardens, on the beach, in the jungle ... Information must come to him full-flavoured from his own observations of native life, and not be squeezed out of reluctant informants as a trickle of talk[2].'

Observational Studies in Nursing

While ethnographic accounts of unfamiliar groups are fascinating, accounts of groups which you think you already understand can be even more so.

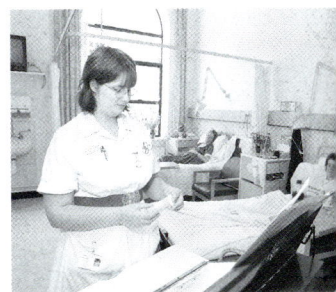

ACTIVITY 2
diary
You already know about nursing because you are a nurse. What value could reading ethnographic accounts of nursing have for you? Write notes in your diary.

FEEDBACK

Ethnographic accounts can offer insights into sub-groups which you know little about. For example, nurses working in the community often know relatively little about current patterns of ward work, and nurses in A&E may know little about the realities of either community or ward work.

Our clients may have encountered more groups of nurses than we have — and their expectations of nursing may have been formed in a different context. Reading ethnographic accounts of clients' attitudes can help us to understand more about how others see different parts of the profession.

Accounts of nursing work which we think we do know about are even more interesting because they provide a new or different perspective on something we know well.

ACTIVITY 3
action
During a period on duty,
try to allocate about 10–15 minutes during
which you can try to think of yourself as a 'stranger'
to what is going on.
Put yourself in the shoes of an ethnographic researcher
and think about the following questions:
• Can I categorise the people I see into different
groups, and if so, how?
• Are any activities being carried out that would be very
strange, and may even cause concern if seen in other
circumstances?
• If I had to adopt one of the roles that I see (for example,
patient, client, nurse) which one would I adopt in order
to find out most about the situation?
• If I could interview only one of the groups of people
identified above about what was going on, which
group would I choose?
• Can I see all that I need to see from here?
Are things going on in rooms or
behind curtains that are
important?

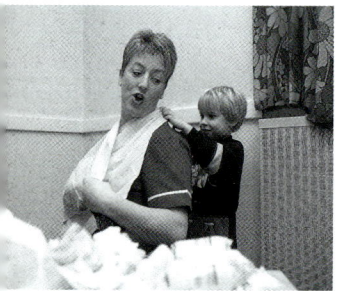

FEEDBACK

Activity 3 should help you to think of some questions to use when reading ethnographic work. For example: 'Could the observer have seen what was going on from there?' 'Would some groups have given biased answers to any questions if they knew the researcher was a nurse?' You may also find it interesting to read *P5: Client Assessment*, and reflect on how some of the discussion about how people's perceptions can affect the information they give might affect the ethnographic collection of data.

ACTIVITY 4
knowledge base
Using your experience as an
ethnographer from the above
Activity, develop a set of
questions with which you could
'interrogate' an ethnographic
research account.
Find an ethnographic account
and test out your list of
questions, adding to it
as necessary.

FEEDBACK

There are no 'right answers' here. You will develop your list as you read more ethnographic work. Particular issues to bear in mind are the gender, age and background of the researchers, and how these factors may affect their status as observer. In Activity 3 you were also asked to think about your informants — the people you would choose to ask questions about what was going on. The type of information you got might well have been different from different groups.

ACTIVITY 5
diary
Make some notes on
how different groups you
observed in Activity 3 might
have given you a different
'story' about a particular
aspect of what was
going on.

Unstructured Interviews

In an ideal world, the ethnographer asks everybody's opinion about everything that is going on. However, in reality, observational studies are time-consuming and expensive, so much ethnographic work today uses extensive *unstructured interviews* rather than observations.

ACTIVITY 6
diary
Read the brief extract alongside, which is taken from a research interview. Note down in your diary how far you think the mother is a suitable person to provide information about:
• Her own thoughts and feelings about the situation
• Martin's thoughts and feelings.

'I: Could I just ask you first to tell me a bit about Martin?

M: Martin is now 24. He's a Down's syndrome and a quiet boy, no trouble at all. He was hyperactive as a child, but he's very easy to get on with, you know. A quiet boy, gentle boy. He loves his food, likes his glass of wine ...

I: Can you tell me, before he went away this last time, had he stayed away from home at all?

M: Oh, he's been away. I used to let him go away for a fortnight almost every year ... That was good for him, it was a leading up over the years. And giving my husband and me a much needed break ...

I: And how did Martin take to going away?

M: Martin loved it ... He loves clubs and, although he's a quiet boy ... he likes company. He's a social lad in a quiet way[3].'

FEEDBACK

The interviewer in this case would probably have found out much more about Martin's mother's view, than about what Martin himself thought. This is fine in ethnography, as long as the researcher is aware of it.

Conversation Analysis

Another type of ethnographic work which is becoming increasingly popular in nursing is *conversation analysis*. This has evolved with the use of very small and easy-to-use tape recorders and video-recorders, which can then be introduced into situations relatively unobtrusively. Audiotape is particularly useful in studying situations where talk is a major activity — health visiting, for example.

The following Activity asks you to do some audio-recording of your own. In using this method, permission must always be sought from the subjects before recording any conversation.

ACTIVITY 7
action
Tape-record a situation from your everyday life, a 10-minute period over supper time for example, or having a drink at the pub. Then play back the tape and write down exactly what was said, including *how* it was said. Include everything — silences, overlaps, repetition, hesitation, and so on.

FEEDBACK

Sometimes we see written down examples of talk, known as transcripts, that are very neat and grammatical. You will have realised from the previous Activity that in real life we do not talk like that — talk is a very 'messy' and very detailed procedure. It is clear from making detailed transcripts, as you did above, that we can respond to events in speech — a silence or a sound — of less than one-tenth of a second. So when reading any research which is based on the analysis of talk, you should consider the detail in the transcripts available to you, and what might have been left out as well as what was included.

We have seen that ethnographers' and phenomenologists' data are largely based on what other people tell them. As we said earlier, surveys also use information given by word of mouth. Yet the two come from totally different traditions of research. So how do these methods differ?

QUALITATIVE AND QUANTITATIVE RESEARCH

The difference between data gathered by surveys in answer to questions and data gathered by ethnographers or phenomenologists in answer to questions really lies in how the answers are analysed.

Although they may both collect data in the form of talk, the survey researcher at some point will translate that talk into a numerical measure. For example, it will become a figure 1 in a box marked Z to be added to all the other figures in the same box.

> **ACTIVITY 8**
> **diary**
> In response to the question 'Do you like custard?' 42 respondents said they did not. List six different ways in which this could have been expressed (for example, 'Custard — yuck!').

Within the survey methodology, all these answers count as the same thing — they are one variable. The respondent either *did* or *did not* like custard. To the phenomenologist, on the other hand, the range of different ways of expressing the answer may itself have been important. This is an illustration of the difference between *quantitative* research (which is based on *numbers* of things) and *qualitative* research, which analyses things by *describing* them.

Many ethnographers are quite comfortable using numbers if it helps their analysis. However, in nursing research there is a tendency towards using qualitative methods of analysing data.

> **ACTIVITY 9**
> **knowledge base**
> Read the account of quantitative analysis alongside. It describes work Silverman did within an ethnographic study of doctor and patient behaviour within oncology clinics[4]. He was particularly concerned to explore differences between NHS clinics and a clinic in the private sector. Underline those aspects of the report which provide qualitative information and those which provide quantitative information.

'My overall impression was that private consultations lasted considerably longer than those held in the NHS clinics. When examined, the data indeed did show that the former were almost twice as long as the latter (20 minutes as against 11 minutes) and that the difference was statistically highly significant (significant at 0.001; $\chi^2 = 69$, 1 d.f.).

'As a further aid to comparative analysis, I measured patient participation in the form of questions and unelicited statements. Once again, a highly significant difference was found: on this measure, private patients participated much more in the consultation (significant at 0.001; $\chi^2 = 22.5$). However, once more taking only patients seen by the same doctor, the difference between the clinics became very small and was not significant (at 0.10). Finally, no significant difference was found in the degree to which non-medical matters (for example, patient's work or home circumstances) were discussed in the clinics.

'These quantitative data were a useful check on over-enthusiastic claims about the degree of difference between the NHS and private clinics. However, it must be remembered that my major concern was with the "ceremonial order" of the three clinics. I had amassed a considerable number of exchanges in which doctors and patients appeared to behave in the private clinic in a manner deviant from what we know about NHS hospital consultations. The question was: would the quantitative data offer any support to my observations?'

In this example, the researcher developed hunches or hypotheses as a result of his observations, and used statistical methods of analysis to test them. Used in this way, the two methodologies work together — neither would have produced a coherent piece of research on its own.

However, there are a number of ways of analysing qualitative data[5] which go beyond reporting anecdotes yet do not resort to presenting numerical statistics. When qualitative results are presented numerically, the richness and impact of the results are often lost. Silverman highlights, in the extract above, that his major concern was with 'ceremonial order' yet the potentially fascinating commentary was lost to statistics.

PICK AND MIX

For the purposes of exploration we have dealt with the methodologies of research separately in the three Parts of R3. However, in the practical world of research they are often combined, as we saw in the example above. The extract below gives an interesting example of research which used fairly standard survey data as well as more unstructured interviews and conversational data.

ACTIVITY 10
knowledge base
Read the extract alongside, and make notes on each type of research method used, which methodology it belongs to, and the criteria you used to identify and categorise each one.
Find another example of a research programme which used a number of methods and more than one approach.

'The information we obtained came from five sources: (a) A questionnaire survey which produced 589 completed questionnaires. 154 came from nurses who had left the employment of the Health Authority in the preceding 15 months; and 435 came from nurses who remained in the employment of the Health Authority . . . A pilot survey for the questionnaire was conducted amongst nurses working in another Health Authority in the same region. (b) 100 nurses were interviewed: 50 were nurses who left during the months of November 1986–January 1987 and 50 were nurses employed by the Health Authority. (c) A cohort of 10 pupil nurses and a cohort of 11 student nurses undertaking general nurse training were interviewed at intervals during their first year. (d) Seven nursing officers were interviewed. (e) Finally, as the research was being carried out, informal conversations and observations were taking place all the time. Such sources of information are important: chance comments lead to new perspectives and redefinitions of the research'[6].

USING RESEARCH

All three parts of *R3: Research Approaches* have explored the different ways in which researchers see the world, and how this affects the way they approach their subject. They consider the methods and methodologies used within the two broad research approaches of positivism and interpretivism.

We have seen that one approach is not necessarily better than another, but that some subjects can be more productively studied within one research tradition than another, and we have tried to identify the sorts of questions that you could ask about any research method to work out how much use the results of that research will be to you in practice.

R4: The Real World of Research looks at some practical issues surrounding how you can implement research findings in practice.

FOCUS

Review your collection of research articles, and use the ideas we have developed over all three Parts of this Section to read each one, and to make sure you are clear about:

- The approach adopted

- The methodology chosen

- The methods used.

Evaluate each of the articles, and write short notes on how useful the findings are to you and to your area of practice.

You should continue to adopt this approach with any research articles you read in the future.

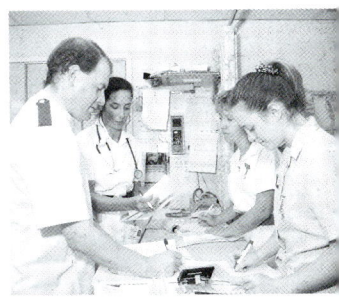

Notes   ## REFERENCES

1   Loftus, L.A. Student nurses' lived experiences of the sudden death of their patients. *Journal of Advanced Nursing* 1998; **27**: 641–648.
2   McNeill, P. *Research Methods*. London: Tavistock, 1985.
3   Richardson, A. 'If you love him, let him go.' In: Brechin, A., Walmsley, J. (eds.). *Making Connections*. London: Hodder and Stoughton, 1989.
4   Silverman, D. *Qualitative Method and Sociology*. London: Gower, 1985.
5   Burnard, P. A Method of analysing interview transcripts in qualitative research. *Nurse Education Today* **11**, 461–466.
6   Mackay, L. *Nursing a Problem*. Milton Keynes: Open University Press, 1989.

FURTHER READING

•   Holloway, I., Wheeler, S. *Qualitative Research for Nurses*. Oxford: Blackwell, 1998.